INTERMITTENT FASTING 16/8

A COMPLETE STEP BY STEP GUIDE TO LOSE WEIGHT EASILY, IMPROVE INSULIN RESISTANCE, OVERALL HEALTH AND LIVE LONGER. A FASTING PROGRAM PERFECT FOR MEN AND WOMEN AND OVER 50

Table of Contents

Introduction

The 16:8 intermittent fasting has become so popular among people over the years. It is because of its many benefits that have helped many people. Intermittent has been shown to help people lose weight and also lower insulin levels and blood sugar. It also has many other benefits, as you will find later in this book.

Intermittent is easy as opposed to what many people think that it is hard. There is little planning required, and many individuals who practice it have said that they feel good generally and more energetic when fasting. When starting, it can be a bit hard, but you get used when the body has adapted.

Throughout this book, you will learn about the 16:8 method of intermittent fasting, how it works, and different foods you can use on this method. The book also has amazingly delicious recipes that are easy to prepare.

Intermittent fasting is different from starvation because you are still eating, just at designated times and sometimes at specific amounts. Fasting can help your body recuperate from the damage of eating food that has poor nutritional values. It can also protect you from sickness and diseases. Fasting, unlike starvation, can clarify your mind and improve organ function, especially regarding the heart. We'll get into the benefits of fasting more within this book.

It's important to note that when using the term "fasting" in this book, we are talking specifically about intermittent fasting, not other kinds. Starting a new fasting program is an exciting time, and we're glad you're reading this book to help you with the process. When you're ready, let's begin!

PART ONE: INTERMITTENT FASTING 16/8 METHOD

Chapter 1: What Is 16/8 Intermittent Fasting?

What is 16:8 Intermittent Fasting?

The 16/8 intermittent fasting protocol for men is among the most successful and widely followed ways to lose weight and gain good health.

You can divide your day into two parts:

- The Fasting Window
- The Eating Window

The best thing about 16/8 intermittent fasting is that it can be made a part of your daily life. It doesn't ask you to do anything extra, and hence, it is easy to follow. There are only two things to be kept in mind.

The hours within which you can eat

The things you should eat

The success of any weight loss plan depends on your dedication to that plan, and intermittent fasting is no exception. Although intermittent fasting puts no holds on the things you can eat and the things you can't. Yet, it is expected of you to show a reasonable attitude towards food items.

You *shouldn't* eat unhealthy things

You *can't* eat stuff in excess quantities

You *mustn't* eat outside your eating window

The Fasting Window

The fasting window should generally begin early in the evening when you are about to finish the active part of the day. There are several benefits to starting the fasting window at the end of the day.

You'd get in the resting mode

Your chances of getting invited to eat something by friends and colleagues would get low

You'd be at a more relaxed atmosphere

Your body would get at least 3-4 hours to digest the food before you hit the bed. Your gut would be grateful for that.

Ideally, the fasting window should begin anywhere between 5-7 in the evening. Men should fast for at least 16 hours, which means if you start your fast around 5 in the evening, you will be able to have the first meal of the day around 9.

If you take it at 7 in the evening, the first meal would not be possible before 11 in the day.

Pushing it any further can keep pushing the first meal of the day farther into the day.

This may not look like a big issue at the moment, but believe me, it's something you should worry about. It takes around 4-5 hours before your gut can properly process a healthy meal; therefore, it is improbable that you would feel any hunger pang before hitting the bed. However, things would be different when you wake up.

Even if you sleep for 7-8 hours, the total fasting time would have been around 12 hours when you wake up. This is the time the hunger starts to build up. If you maintain a healthy exercise routine, you wouldn't feel very hungry for another 1-2 hours as physical activity suppresses the feeling of hunger momentarily. However, the hunger would start building up pretty strongly after that.

I am assuming that you would also need to go to work. Passing the next one or two hours in the fasted state while working can be difficult. Therefore, it is always best to begin the fasting window early, so that you can get the first meal of the day before you start the active part of the day.

Begin your fasting window as early as possible, and try to make it a routine.

Don't shift the timings a lot as your body would also need to adjust to the routine

It is important that you somewhat fix the timings of your first and last meal of the day

Eating Window

You get 8 hours for the eating window. These 8 hours are important as you will need to take all the nutrition during these

8 hours. It may look like a lot of time, but it isn't. After 16 hours of fasting, when you have the first meal of the day, it is generally complicated to have another meal after 4 hours.

You will also need to ensure that you don't indulge in overeating.

If you don't have a properly balanced meal, transitioning from one meal to another smoothly without the urge to have something in between will become difficult.

Therefore, you must have a very balanced first meal of the day.

It should have all the macronutrients and should provide the required minerals and vitamins that your body needs.

The first meal of the day is crucial as it is going to be the most fulfilling meal for you. It is always best that you get it at home. You get complete control over the ingredients of your meal, and the way you prepare it. If you have your meals out, you can't be sure of these things.

You must always remember that food is a significant part of any weight-loss strategy; therefore, you can't ignore this part completely.

Although you can have three meals in the 8 hours eating window, it is generally not possible to have three proper meals in this short gap. If you have a healthy and fulfilling meal at the start of the day, you are not likely to have the urge to have a complete meal at lunch.

The lunch should be light, as it can make you feel lethargic. Generally, the last meal of the day is the second proper meal you will be able to have, and that's why you will have to focus on the first and last meal.

Exercise

Exercise is another important part of an intermittent fasting routine. Intermittent fasting helps your body in getting into the fat-burning mode. However, it is your job to create the energy demand. If you are leading a highly active life, then that can come naturally, but the chances of the same are slim. This makes it important that you create the energy demands through exercise.

High-Intensity Interval Training is one of the best ways to create high energy demands quickly. It pushes your body to burn calories faster. Intermittent fasting also leads to an increase in the production of HGH in your body and also helps increase your fat-burning abilities through exercise.

You will need to remain in the fasted state for at least 16 hours in a day to get the maximum benefits.

The longer you would fast, the better the results would be.

You should try to extend the fasting hours as much as possible.

The best strategy to do so would be to begin the fasting early and start pushing the breakfast later into the day.

You should reduce the intake of refined carbs and sugar in your diet.

You should also reduce your reliance on processed food items as much as possible.

The shift towards the whole and unprocessed food items.

Drink plenty of fluids.

You can have unsweetened black tea and coffee, and even fresh lime water for suppressing the hunger pangs.

However, you should avoid excessive consumption of tea or coffee in both the fasting as well as eating windows.

You must take as much rest as possible.

Sleeping for at least 7-8 hours is very important for faster weight loss.

On this intermittent fasting method, you fast 16 hours of the day and only eat during the remaining 8 hours of the day. The fasting window is a total of 16 hours a day; Your fasting window will mostly be during the time you are sleeping. During your fasting window, you will not eat any calories at all. Not eating when your mind and body are accustomed to eating will be difficult, but the challenge is mind over matter, and you matter so you will succeed. Choose a time to start and stop your feeding window, when the feeding window stops, the fasting window starts, and when the fasting window stops, the feeding window starts, and so on.

People who Cannot Fast on the Plan

Intermittent Fasting can work for anyone. It can help anyone get healthy, lose weight, and build lean muscles. However, there are a few exceptions. These exceptions are mainly for safety and health reasons. Certain current health conditions may worsen when you enter long fasting periods.

Sleep-deprived or stressed

People who are experiencing high-stress levels for quite a long time are not good candidates for long fasting periods. These also include those who are sleep-deprived. Sleep deprivation and chronic high-stress levels take a huge toll on health. Add fasting periods, and the body will be subjected to extremely high strain. This can seriously deplete the body's capability to compensate and keep the organs working, further leading to a host of severe, potentially fatal conditions. There can be accelerated cell aging and death, accumulation of toxins, reduced immunity and slowing of metabolism and organ functioning.

It is advisable to address stress and sleep deprivation first before going into the IF lifestyle.

Sugar or food addict

If you have an addiction to sugar or certain food, fasting will become especially challenging. You will experience intensified cravings. If you are trying to wean off sugar, then fasting may cause you to relapse. There is a huge possibility that you will gorge on high sugar foods during the eating window. It is better to find other ways to deal with sugar addiction.

Pregnant and breastfeeding women, children

These people have high nutritional requirements for various metabolic and growth needs. Pregnant women need to eat to provide for the nutritional needs of the baby. Prolonged fasting states in pregnant women can lead to weakness and some potential complications like poor fetal growth.

For breastfeeding women, long fasting periods are also not recommended. They need to eat because they have to retain a good supply of nutrients for breast milk production. They also need the energy to replenish what they lost during the milk production process and the breastfeeding sessions. This stage can be really taxing on a woman's strength.

Children are at a stage of rapid growth and development. They have high nutritional requirements to fuel growth spurt and the maturation of their various organs. This is not the time to force their bodies to rely on fat stores during fasted states. It is still better for children to eat nutritious foods whenever they are hungry.

People with Medical and Mental Illness

So, the first mental illness we're going to cover is eating disorders because they are all about what you eat and how you think about food. They can be challenging to overcome. Generally, there are three eating disorders: anorexia, bulimia, and binge eating. All of these represent difficulty with food and the person's relationship with food. Anorexia and fasting should not mix. Anorexia is, essentially, starvation and results in significant malnourishment. If you have a history of anorexia, you shouldn't fast. Starting a fast can cause you to relapse into anorexia instead of keeping a healthy eating/resting schedule. If you experience bulimia and binging, you also should not be fasting. Again, all these eating disorders represent a misunderstanding of the purpose of food to our health and well-being. Fasting restricts what you eat and can cause you to relapse into an eating disorder if you already have a history of one. So please do not pursue fasting if you previously had an eating disorder.

Advanced Diabetes

While fasting can help with insulin resistance, if you already have diabetes, then fasting isn't for you. You shouldn't pursue it until after talking with your doctor. Fasting can cause changes in your insulin levels, metabolic levels, and of course, your glucose levels. This can play life-endangering havoc with your body if you are already struggling with insulin and hormone levels. Please, please, please, speak to your doctor before even approaching fasts. Your doctor will be able to give you a better idea of your body's current state and where you can adjust with your eating without fasting.

Irritable Bowel Syndrome

If you have irritable bowel syndrome, fasting isn't recommended. This is because fasting can impact the way you digest food and how your metabolism works. This can cause some irritation to an already-irritable bowel. Some people have experienced bloating while fasting as well. So, speak with your doctor about what you can do with fasting before starting.

In general, if you have a medical condition, you should speak with your doctor before starting any new diet or fast. Your doctor knows what your body can handle, and they can give you recommendations for meeting your dietary goals without risking your health.

Children

It's so easy to be a child or a teenager and feel pressure to look like celebrities do. Girls especially have been taught they have to look away within our society. They may look through social media and find many examples of the perfect body. They may want that body for themselves and choose to control their food and their relationship to food by dieting. However, this is an easy way to slip into disordered eating. Children shouldn't fast. Full stop. Children are using each piece of food they eat to grow and develop their bodies and brains. They are creating a system that works for them, but also creating habits that can be lifelong. Fasting can easily slip into anorexia. It's an easy slope to fall, and children are still learning about their relationship with food and how it makes them feel. If they fast, they may learn to make it a habit that can lead to poor nutrition or even disordered eating, all of which can persist within their adult lives. Children shouldn't fast. If your child or teenager wants to improve their diet, they can do that by choosing healthy options for food, having nutritious meals, and exercising. They don't need to fast to achieve their diet and body goals, and they shouldn't.

Why Should You Choose 16:8 Fasting?

The 16/8 Intermittent Fasting protocol is particularly attractive for beginner fasters for a good reason.

While most other programs tend to impose upon you a very restrictive set of dietary rules, the 16/8 program doesn't do any of that!

This is a very simple and easy to follow diet program and will allow you to bring in awesome results with minimal effort.

Due to the versatility and flexibility of the protocol, it is rather easy for any individual to squeeze this program into their daily lifestyle seamlessly.

 In addition to helping you to lose weight, the 16/8 program also will help you to improve your cranial functionality, improve your sugar levels, and increase your overall longevity.

So, if this is your first time trying fast, the 16/8 is possibly the perfect and best option for you!

And even if you are fasting veteran, the 16/8 will also help you to wind down a bit from your more hardcore fasting programs while still being able to enjoy the benefits of fasting.

Side Effects of the 16/8 Intermittent Fasting

While intermittent fasting is one of the most beneficial eating patterns that you can try at present, you still need to be extremely cautious before starting. Keep in mind that it is not risk-free. This makes it necessary to talk to your physician first and find out whether it is safe for you to follow this style of eating.

Also, find out if you have any health problems or complications that might cause the negative side effects, instead of rewarding benefits, of intermittent fasting to come out. It also helps to understand the most common side effects of intermittent fasting so you can study the whole approach carefully and find out how you can avoid them as much as possible.

Tiredness – When doing IF, there is a high risk for you to experience tiredness and grogginess, especially if you are still a beginner. Take note that in this situation, your body will also most likely run on less energy than what it is used to. Fasting might also increase your stress level and disrupt your standard sleep patterns. To avoid this specific side effect of intermittent fasting, it would be helpful for you to meditate or do other activities that will lower your stress levels. If you are working out regularly, then consider scheduling it during your eating period. This helps conserve your energy. Also, keep in mind that exercising while you are on the fasted state might lower your blood sugar level, which can trigger symptoms, like confusion and dizziness. It helps to be on the safe side by working out when you have already eaten.

Headaches – You may be dealing with headaches because your body will tend to adjust to your new eating pattern. It could be caused by dehydration, so it is advisable to drink plenty of water both during your eating window and fasting period. You may also experience headaches due to a sudden drop in your blood sugar level and the release of stress hormones during the fasting period. The good news is that headaches usually happen only because your body is still on the adjustment stage. This means that this side effect is not permanent. Once you get used to it, you will no longer suffer from headaches.

Heartburn – You may also experience heartburn due to fasting. In most cases, this problem will be resolved after around a couple of months. It is necessary to visit and consult your doctor in case your heartburn does not seem to resolve on its own even after your body has adjusted to the new eating pattern. Heartburn is often a result of your unfamiliarity to the fasting scenario, causing your body to release stomach acids automatically at certain times. While this can cause discomfort, this only happens at the beginning of your journey, so there is no need for you to worry too much about it.

Brain fog – This is also another common side effect of intermittent fasting, especially if your body is not yet used to the habit of not eating. This might cause your mind to try keeping up with the new routine, leading to confusion, forgetfulness, or brain fog. Once you familiarize yourself with how IF works, though, and your body has adjusted to the habit, you can expect better brain function from fasting.

Diarrhea – Another unpleasant side effect of IF is diarrhea, and it usually happens to those who are still beginners in fasting. There is an even higher risk for you to experience this problem if you enter the fasting period after consuming too many carbs. This problem may be associated with a significant drop in your insulin level, signaling your kidneys to get rid of excess water. This is the reason why you might experience unwanted and watery bowel movements. You should also remember that your body tends to lose electrolytes via bowel movements and urination. If you experience watery stools or diarrhea, then one sign that you may experience at first is a low level of sodium. With that in mind, it helps to drink broth or pickle juice during those days when you are dealing with this uncomfortable and unwanted IF side effect. It also helps to add around 1-2 pinches of salt in the water you drink.

Insomnia and anxiety – Both these side effects may be caused by the production of adrenaline, a counter-regulatory hormone when you begin to fast. In most cases, this effect is actually beneficial as it results in a high metabolic rate and energy level. The problem is that the energy you get from it might be too high even during those specific times when you are supposed to be sleeping. This can also make you feel jittery and anxious. It could be because of consuming too much coffee, especially during the beginning of your fasting journey. Your anxiety also tends to worsen if you constantly worry about the effects of fasting on your health. You can resolve these side effects by sticking to proper bedtime routines, such as turning off your gadgets and electronics ninety minutes before your bedtime. You can also relax with the help of Epsom salt baths.

Bad breath – Another unpleasant and unexpected side effect of intermittent fasting is bad breath. This often happens if you already start losing weight due to fasting. This side effect is also referred to as the keto breath characterized by your tongue becoming white and a taste of acetone in your mouth. It is mainly because acetone is known as the by-product of metabolizing fatty acid. A lot of those who tried fasting and experienced the keto breath tend to freak out upon noticing their white tongues. They even wrongly assume that it is a result of nutrient deficiency. If this happens to you, then avoid freaking out. This is your body's normal reaction to the fat-burning process. As weight loss starts slowing down, you will notice a great improvement in your breath. You will also notice your tongue going back to its normal pink color. If you feel uncomfortable with this side effect, then there are some things that you can do to manage it. One is to brush your teeth as frequently as possible throughout the day. Drinking more water and using a tongue scraper can also help. Intermittent fasting provides numerous benefits to those who are obese, overweight and have average weight. However, it is not appropriate for everyone, including pregnant and breastfeeding women and those who are dealing with eating disorders and certain health issues.

This is the main reason why you have to study the effects of fasting to you as soon as you begin doing it. Listen to your own body. If you notice some unwanted side effects, find out if it is because your body is just adjusting to the routine or due to more serious issues. If you are extremely worried about the negative side effects, do not hesitate to consult your doctor to ensure your safety.

How the 16:8 IF Diet Works

In this method of IF, you only eat within 8 hours and then fast for 16 hours. Most people will think that this will cause them to experience extreme hunger. Normally, we eat all day - from the time we get up in the morning and until we finally go to sleep at night. That will be averaging anywhere from 12 to 14 hours. This is called the fed state.

In this state, the body focuses more on digesting and absorbing recently eaten foods. These processes can take up to several hours. During the fed state, the body's fat-burning processes are at a minimum. It is hard for the body to burn stored fats during the fed state because it relies on the energy derived from recent food consumption.

Insulin levels are high during the fed state. This is a response to the influx of glucose from foods. This more elevated insulin level also hinders fat burning.

After the fed state, the body enters the post-absorptive state. In this state, the body is neither digesting nor processing food. This usually lasts for about 1 to 2 hours after you last ate a meal.

After the post-absorptive state, if you still haven't eaten or drank anything that contains calories, your body enters the fasted state.

During the fasting period, your digestive system does not actively digest solid foods. Instead, it concentrates on fully metabolizing and absorbing the nutrients from foods. This becomes an opportunity to utilize foods fully and turn these into readily usable energies. This energy is quickly used up by the body. Efficient energy use lessens the possibility of converting excess calories into fats.

In the fasted state, levels of insulin are low. The inhibitory effect of insulin on fat-burning is reduced; hence, the body can turn on its fat-burning processes at full force. This is why people who go on intermittent fasts burn fats and lose weight without changing their current diet. Even if they still eat the same kinds of foods every day, weight loss is evident.

Steady weight loss is achievable in the 8:16 intermittent fasting diet. This is because the cells burn glycogen stores for energy during the fasted state. When you eat again to break the fast, your body will turn energy into glycogen, instead of turning it into fat cells. This further enhances weight maintenance by reducing the amount of food that gets turned and stored as fats.

If you're eating for two, you should not be skipping meals. Unless your doctor says that you must fast, please don't. At this stage of your health and your baby's development, you need to take the right balance of nutrients and calories. Fasting can mess with this. Beyond this, while pregnant, there are often vitamins and additional medications that need to be taken. Many of these need to be taken with food. Fasting can make this difficult. Finally, with pregnancy comes hormone changes. Fasting also causes some hormone changes (as mentioned in the section about circadian rhythm). You don't want to be adding additional stress to your body because it's already changing to accommodate the baby. So please don't fast until your baby is weaned, and you're both happy and healthy.

How to Follow The 16:8 Method

The 16:8 method is very flexible, and that means you can choose your own specific 8-hour eating window, according to your day. You might work shifts, and that means you sleep at different times. What you should do in that case is pick an 8-hour window, which is when you are mostly awake. Obviously!

For example, if you are working nights and you are sleeping between the hours of 10 am and 6 pm, that means you can eat from 6 pm until 2 am. You would then probably be working until the following morning when you would head off to sleep, but you could drink coffee (unsweetened and black) to keep you going also, and plenty of water. This might not work for you, so you could think about shifting your pattern and starting it later, perhaps if you don't feel like eating the moment you open your eyes. You could then choose an eating window of 9 pm and eat freely until 5 am.

It's really up to you!

We've already covered the two main methods most people try with the 16:8, and that is the skipping breakfast and starting to eat at lunchtime routine, or in the case of someone who really needs breakfast because they can't concentrate without it.

It's not only about when you can eat, but it's also about what you eat too. Whilst there are no restrictions and no lists of foods you must eat and foods you shouldn't, always remember that if you suddenly pile a huge breakfast or lunch on your plate after fasting, you're going to end up with stomach ache. That could mean that you end up eating too many calories within your eating window and put weight on, or you end up with stomach disturbances for the rest of your eating window, don't get enough fuel during that time because your stomach is so bloated you can't bear to eat, and then you're hungry during your fasting time. It's about choosing carefully, which we'll talk about a little more shortly.

So, how many calories should you eat? It depends on whether you want to lose weight or maintain. A standard calorie amount to maintain weight is 2500 calories per day for a man and 2000 calories per day for a woman. This does depend on the height, current weight, and metabolism of the person, and is only an average, healthy amount. If you want more solid guidelines on your specific circumstances, speak to your doctor, who will be able to give you a calorie aim plan tailored to your needs.

Within that calorie amount, you should make sure that you get a good, varied diet. That means proteins, carbs, fats, vitamins, and minerals. Again, we're going to cover what you can and can't eat, loosely because there are no rules, shortly, but varied is the way to go. Ironically this will also help you enjoy your new lifestyle more because you're not bored and eating the same things all the time. This is a pitfall many people suffer from regular low-calorie diets; the change is so restrictive that they end up eating the same thing day in, day out, and over time they get so bored and simply rebel against it. This usually ends in a binge day, which causes extreme guilt and then leads them to throw the diet in the bin and go back to eating whatever they want.

Whilst following the 16:8 method, you should also make sure that you drink plenty of water throughout the day, whether fasting or eating. This ensures that you don't become dehydrated and will also aid in digestion. Besides, you should also exercise too!

Now, there are no rules to say that you must exercise whilst following an intermittent fasting routine, but it will help you lose weight faster, and it will help with your general health and well-being. Exercise is fantastic on so many levels, not least helping to build lean muscle, which also boosts your ability to burn fat as an energy source. Exercise is also known to help with mental health issues, such as anxiety and depression, as well as stress. We all live stressful lives, and a little exercise can sometimes be enough to reduce it to extremely manageable levels. Aside from anything else, exercise can be a sociable and fun activity!

Why Is It Hard Stay On a Diet?

Oftentimes, we find ourselves stuck in our efforts to lose weight. Last year you tried to lose weight, but nothing changed. This is what happened the year before last year. So, you are still not sure whether you will make this the year to change. We all have gone through a similar experience. Without a doubt, it is frustrating to make plans to lose weight, and yet nothing ever seems to change. Most people end up giving up.

The idea of losing weight is not as easy as it sounds. In fact, it is far easier said than done. It is very easy for you to say that you will begin eating the right foods and exercise regularly. However, when you wake up the following morning, your plans will have gone out of the window. The next thing you know, you're waking up late, gaining more weight, and cursing yourself.

But why is it so difficult to stay on a diet? Of course, we know the negative effects of eating junk food and other unhealthy meals. Regardless, we still find ourselves eating these foods. This means that we eat unhealthy foods regularly in spite of their associated negative effects. This leaves us with the question - why is it so hard to stick to a diet? Why is it difficult for people to stay away from something they know will have a negative impact on their health?

The Stomach vs. The Brain

Logically, there is a good reason why people eat food. Eating food provides the body with the required energy to function optimally. It is through eating that the body can effectively store energy for later use. Also, our food intake ensures that the body obtains the right nutrients to facilitate growth and maintain its regular functioning. Consequently, the digestive system is a complex system capable of functioning on its own to monitor and gauge what we consume.

To understand how the human brain has changed what goes into our stomachs, consider our cravings for spicy foods. Eating spicy foods causes pain. However, this is what people like. But, often, you will come across people saying "Great, I love that." Why do you think this happens?

Even though the digestive system knows what the body needs, the brain seems to have taken over. It acts as a manager that determines what we should eat. So, could this be the main reason why folks are pushed to engage in binge eating regardless of its associated negative effects?

Well, the way in which the brain functions to determine what we should eat makes logical sense. It drives us to eat what we should not be eating. Instead of reducing our food quantities, we continue eating more. Think about it this way: after eating a heavy meal during lunch hour, why is it that you cannot resist dessert? How the human brain affects our decisions is to be blamed. If the digestive system could decide for us, then, of course, you would not want to eat more because you would already be full.

Clearly, our diet is controlled by the digestive system and the brain in tandem. However, the two systems can't get along peacefully. Since the two can't agree on anything, it leaves us with a burden of managing what we should eat. Consequently, with stress mounting on our shoulders, we are simply forced to eat. The cycle continues, and for that reason, we find it difficult to stay on a diet.

Choosing the Wrong Diet

Let's not put the blame wholly on the brain. Another reason why you might be a diet-failure is because of selecting the wrong diet in the first place. Dieting should mean that you change what you eat completely. You should bear in mind that you are trying to change a habit you have been accustomed to for years now. Consequently, coming up with a new list of what you should eat will not make sense. Your diet plan should be reasonable. It should feature a few things you love to eat and other foods that will have a positive impact on your weight loss plan.

Dieting Without Exercise

Your dieting failure could also be as a result of your lack of exercise. It is recommended that you diet while at the same time working out. Regular exercise will not only bring health benefits your way, but it will also help you psychologically. Therefore, your mind will be healthy enough to focus on what you want to achieve.

Failing to Change Your Environment

Sure, you might have the willpower to follow a diet plan. Nevertheless, if you fail to change your environment, it will be difficult for you to focus. The environment where you are should be diet-friendly. This means that it should not be full of foods that can easily tempt you. The last thing that you need as you try to fast is to deal with temptations. Simply ensure that your environment is friendly enough. If you have family members who will make it difficult for you to fast, then there is a high chance that it will be a challenge for you to meet your goals.

Using an Unsustainable Plan

One of the main reasons why it is difficult to follow a certain diet plan is because the plan is unsustainable. Yes, your plan can work, but it is not practical. For instance, the fact that you want to lose weight doesn't necessarily mean that you should stay away from fats completely. When creating a diet plan, you have to consider whether you can live with the plan for the next year or so. If not, then it is highly likely that you might drop it after a week.

Your diet plan should be not only easy to follow, but also flexible. Starting your diet plan with strict measures will only affect you negatively. You will be stressed out every time you realize that you didn't achieve your goals. Equally, your plan should never be a way of keeping you away from the foods you like. Frankly, there are diet plans whereby you lose weight while still eating your favorite dishes.

Therefore, staying on a diet plan might seem impossible because your strategy is not sustainable. It is important that you adopt a plan that you can work with for more than six months.

Over Indulging With Food

From a general perspective, the relationship that you have with food will have a huge impact on whether or not you lose weight. We all know of those individuals who strive to lose weight, and yet they switch foods. One month they stick to a particular food choice, and the following month they are trying something else. If you fall under this category, then you cannot lose weight in the long run. Eventually, it will be difficult for you to lose weight, and this will discourage you.

One thing you don't realize is that you are only changing what you are eating. However, you are not changing the relationship you have with food. It is crucial that you learn how to tune your mindset to relate in a particular manner with food. Changing your mindset helps a lot, more so in the long run. You will not indulge in unhealthy eating habits in the future as you know your limits. Also, your mind is fully aware of the benefits you are looking to get through your food choices.

Guidelines for Intermittent 16:8

Now that the basics of the 16/8 protocol are covered, let me walk you through how you can actually start following the program.

I have already laid down the ground rules of the program, so let's dig deep.

So, the first step for you to do is to choose your fasting window.

We already know that you need to fast for 8 hours, right? So let's talk about that.

Many people opt to eat between the noontime and 8 pm, this allows individuals to cut a good chunk of fasting time, and after the last meal, they can just go to sleep.

Afterward, you can simply have a balanced and healthy dinner and lunch to maintain your daily calorie intake.

On the other hand, some people tend to eat between 9 am and 5 pm, which will give you enough time to have a healthy breakfast at around 9 am, have a fine lunch at noon, a light dinner or snack at around 4 pm and finally start your fasting for 8 hours.

But the above mentioned two were just simple examples; you are allowed to choose your very own plan as you need.

You should keep in mind though that during your "Eating" window, you must prevent yourself from overeating; otherwise, nothing will work out.

The meals and snacks should be spaced out properly in order to help your body adjust to your blood sugar levels and appetite.

Also, if you want to enhance the effectiveness of this program further, you should try to stick to unprocessed "whole" food and healthy beverages.

A good way to deal with this is to balance out your meals by having meals that include ingredients such as:

·   Poultry, fish, meat, eggs, nuts, seeds, etc. for protein

·   Coconut oil, avocados, olive oil as your healthy fat

·   Rice, oats, barley, buckwheat, quinoa as your healthy fats

·   Tomatoes, leafy greens, cucumber, broccoli, cauliflower, etc. as your veggies

·   Orange, apple, bananas, berries, peaches, pears as healthy fruits

During your fasting periods, you are allowed to go for simple calorie-free beverages such as water or even unsweetened coffee or tea, and they will help you stay hydrated and control your appetite.

And as mentioned earlier, if you eat more and more junk food, then all the positive effects of the 16/8 program will be negated, and it might ultimately do more harm to your health than good.

To summarize, this particular protocol of Intermittent Fasting is really easy to get into and is a hassle-free way of experiencing how fasting works if you haven't already.

Plus, it gives enough feeding time so that you don't feel incredibly weak and allows your body to slowly adjust itself to the physiological and cellular changes that are accompanied by the protocol and fasting itself.

Typical Schedule for the 16/8 method

We've gone over the step-by-step process of transitioning into your fast. We've also looked a bit at making sure you have a clear record of the steps you are taking and how your body is adapting to the fast. Now let's look at some possible schedules for your fast. There is a schedule for your transition period and a schedule that examines what your daily eating times and windows will look like. Here are some additional things to keep in mind before looking at schedules:

• Your choice of schedule is personal. Create one based on your work schedule or other circumstances in your life. If you want to have dinner with your family, then use that meal to close out your eating window. Count back eight hours to figure out when your first meal will be.

• Your fasting schedule doesn't have to be set in stone. Try out different times or change your fasting window for special occasions. You don't want to be limited by your schedule, especially when it comes to your social life.

• A great option for scheduling is to follow the times when you're naturally more awake and aware and end your fast before your natural slumps. Each person has a different internal clock, so determine your schedule based on that. Following your natural circadian rhythm is a good place to start; adapt from there.

Early Eating Schedule

This schedule is a great option because it takes advantage of your circadian rhythm. It also is the ideal time in general to eat because it avoids eating late at night. However, it means that you're going to eat an early dinner, which might not work for everyone. With this schedule, you'll start eating at 7:00 am and end at 3:00 pm.

Here is how to ease into your fast:

Time	Days 1–3	Days 4–6	Days 7–9	Days 10–12
7:00 a.m.	Wake up Eat	Wake up Eat	Wake up Eat	Wake up Eat
9:00 a.m.				
11:00 a.m.	Eat	Eat	Eat	Eat

1:00 p.m.				
3:00 p.m.	Snack		Eat	Eat before 3
5:00 p.m.		Eat	Fast	Fast
7:00 p.m.	Eat	Fast	Fast	Fast
9:00 p.m.	Fast	Fast	Fast	Fast
10:00 p.m.	Sleep/fast	Sleep/fast	Sleep/fast	Sleep/fast

Here is your weeklong schedule once you've eased into the fast:

Time	12:00 a.m.– 7:00 a.m.	7:00 a.m.	11:00 a.m.	2:00 p.m.	3:00 p.m.– 2:00 a.m.
Monday to Sunday	Fast/sleep	Breakfast (either light or the largest meal of the day)	Large meal	Last meal, finished by 3:00 p.m.	Fast/sleep

Midday Eating Schedule

Some people have difficulty with eating first thing in the morning. In this case, you can start your fast later in the day. This fast is ideal for people who want to eat right in the middle of the day. It gives you time to wind down before bed and prepare your body for a time of rest without too much digestion happening while you sleep. It also gives you time to exercise in the morning before you break your fast if you want to.

Here is how to ease into your fast:

Time	Days 1–3	Days 4–6	Days 7–9	Days 10–12
6:00 a.m.	Sleep/eat	Sleep/east	Sleep/fast	Sleep/fast
8:00 a.m.	Eat	Eat	Eat	Fast
10:00 a.m.				Eat
12:00 p.m.	Eat	Eat	Eat	
2:00 p.m.	Snack	Snack		Eat
4:00 p.m.				

6:00 p.m.	Eat	Eat	Eat	Eat before 6:00 p.m.
8:00 p.m.			Fast	Fast
10:00 p.m.	Sleep/fast	Sleep/fast	Sleep/fast	Sleep/fast

Here is your weeklong schedule once you've eased into the fast:

Time	12:00 a.m.–7:00 a.m.	10:00 a.m.	2:00 p.m.	5:00 p.m.	6:00 p.m.–12:00 a.m.
Monday to Sunday	Fast/sleep	Breakfast (either light or the largest meal of the day)	Large meal	Last meal finished by 6:00 p.m.	Fast/sleep

Evening Eating Schedule

This schedule doesn't take advantage of your circadian rhythm, and it might not give you the most benefits in changing glucose and cortisol levels. However, this schedule can work for people who really appreciate social eating or people who work at unconventional hours. You can always eat a bit earlier to change this schedule.

Here is how to ease into your fast:

Time	Days 1–3	Days 4–6	Days 7–9	Days 10–12
12:00 a.m.–6:00 a.m.	Sleep/fast	Sleep/fast	Sleep/fast	Sleep/fast
8:00 a.m.	Fast	Fast	Fast	Fast
10:00 a.m.	Eat	Fast	Fast	Fast
12:00 p.m.		Eat	Fast	Fast
2:00 p.m.	Eat		Eat	Fast
4:00 p.m.	Snack	Eat	Snack	Eat
6:00 p.m.		Snack		
8:00 p.m.	Eat		Eat	Eat

10:00 p.m.		Eat		
12:00 a.m.			Eat	Eat before midnight

Here is your weeklong schedule once you've eased into the fast:

Time	12:00 a.m.– 8:00 a.m.	8:00 a.m.– 4:00 p.m.	4:00 p.m.	8:00 p.m.	11:00 p.m.– 12:00 a.m.
Monday to Sunday	Fast/sleep	Fast	Breakfast (either light or the largest meal of the day)	Large meal	Last meal, finished by midnight

These three different schedules give you some options for following your 16/8 fasting schedule. As mentioned before, adapt the programs to fit your daily rhythm and lifestyle better. It's ideal if your schedule is consistent, but it doesn't have to be set in stone. If you know you want to celebrate your best friend's promotion at the end of the week, then shift your fasting schedule to accommodate eating with your friends. Remember, fasting isn't a diet; it's just an eating schedule. It doesn't need to be permanent, and there shouldn't be any guilt about shifting your schedule. Since we've now discussed several schedule possibilities and how to ease into them, we'll spend the next couple of chapters looking at food choices and some meal plans.

Chapter 2: The Benefits of 16:8 Intermittent Fasting

Intermittent fasting techniques, including the 16:8 method, are most commonly used to assist in weight loss by the general population. The method has been tried by thousands of people and also scientifically proven to be a helpful resource in reducing body fat and improving body composition. Weight loss is often considered the number one reason why people opt for a diet and program that utilizes intermittent fasting.

While a reduction in body fat is definitely one of the best advantages to be mentioned in terms of intermittent fasting, there are more advantages that people gain when they decide that they are going to follow this type of program – especially if they truly commit to it and can implement self-control that ensures they do not give in to cravings.

Intermittent fasting is known to assist in improving your body composition as well, as I mentioned earlier. Body composition refers to a series of features – this includes your body fat percentage and lean muscle mass primarily. A program that utilizes intermittent fasting, along with an appropriate diet plan, will bring down your body fat percentage, and push up your lean muscle mass at the same time.

It is also important to note the benefits that are associated with weight loss for people with an excessive amount of fat distributed throughout their bodies. Since overweight and obesity are linked to so many chronic conditions that can truly make your life dreadful, losing even small amounts of weight can drastically reduce your risk of these diseases. Additionally, if you already have a diagnosis of a condition associated with obesity, reduced body weight may improve the symptoms you are experiencing and help you get the disease under control.

Take type 2 diabetes, for example. In one study, scientists describe that factors such as pro-inflammatory markers, cytokines, hormones, glycerol, and no esterified fatty acids are all increased among those people who are obese. In turn, these factors all have factors that link them to insulin resistance. When insulin resistance develops, it can continue to progress into type 2 diabetes if the affected person does not implement appropriate preventative measures.

When you develop type 2 diabetes, you become predisposed to many additional risks and complications. In fact, type 2 diabetes can cause severe complications that may not only lead to disability but also become life-threatening. This disease can also affect all of the body's most important organs, including the heart, and can damage various tissues, such as nerves, throughout the body.

In addition to assisting in reducing body weight and bringing down the risks associated with obesity, intermittent fasting has many other benefits that are also worth mentioning.

Through intermittent fasting, cellular changes may occur in the body. This can lead to levels of human growth hormones rising by as much as 500%. This leads to a faster rate of fat burning while also producing an increase in muscle mass.

It has also been found that intermittent fasting can help to remove waste that has built up in cells within the human body and can also assist in the repair process of cells that have been damaged. This means cells in the body become more efficient in performing their specialized functions.

One study also explains how recent findings from scientists suggest that intermittent fasting helps to improve brain health and may play a crucial role in assisting medical experts to understand better how diseases like Parkinson's disease and Alzheimer's disease can be prevented in the future.

Furthermore, following an intermittent fasting plan can also help to reduce levels of inflammation within the human body, as well as help to fight against oxidative stress. Both of these factors are known to contribute to numerous chronic diseases significantly and can causes certain molecules to become damaged, which can inhibit their functionality within the body.

In one study, scientists tested how intermittent fasting would work on brain health and cardiovascular health among a group of laboratory rats. They found significant improvements in various tests used to determine the well-being of these two crucial hormones of the body. The scientists also associated these improvements among the tested laboratory rats with a reduction in oxidative stress that was observed. Additionally, the scientists also found an increase in the cellular stress resistance ratings in these rats. What this means is that an intermittent fasting diet can help to reduce the effect that stress has on the body, and help to fight against the existing oxidative damage, often also referred to as free radical damage that has already occurred.

It Modulates the Cells, Hormones and Genes Function

The failure to eat for a while leads to certain things happening to the body. For instance, it will start to regulate cell function and change some of your hormone levels, making it easier for body fat to enter. Other changes that may occur in the body include:

Levels of insulin: insulin levels will decline slightly, which makes it easier for the body to burn fat.

Human Growth Hormone: Growth hormone blood level can significantly increase. High levels of this hormone can help build muscle and burn fat.

Cell Repair: The body will begin the process of repairing the cells, such as removing the waste from all the cells

Genetic profiling: Some beneficial mutations occur in several genes that will help you live longer and protect against disease.

Weight Loss and Body Fat

Many people go fast in succession to lose weight. In most cases, intermittent fasting will naturally help you eat less. You will end up consuming fewer calories, which will lead to weight loss. Besides, fasting strengthens the hormone to facilitate weight loss. Low growth hormone and insulin levels help your body break down fat and use energy. This is why short-term fasting can increase your metabolism by at least three percent.

On the one hand, it boosts your metabolism to burn more calories while also reducing the amount you eat. According to a review that was released in 2014concerning the scientific studies of intermittent fasting, people were able to lose up to 8 percent of their body weight in less than 24 weeks.

It Helps with Diabetes

Type 2 diabetes is a disease that has become popular in recent years. Anything that could lower the resistance of insulin could also be useful in reducing the blood sugar levels hence protecting you from type 2 diabetes.

According to some researches on Intermittent Fasting, there was a reduction of blood sugar from three to six percent, while insulin was reduced by 21 percent and 31 percent. A study carried on rats that were diabetic also proved that Intermittent Fasting could be crucial in the protection of rats from kidney damage, a common challenge for diabetics. This suggests that indirect fasting may be a good option for people at high risk for type 2 diabetes.

Simplifying Life

While this may not be considered a health benefit like any other, it is still important to note. Many people find that temporary fasting can make life easier. They know that they need to have a focus on to eat, as long as they are allowed to eat for hours. They can go a few days a week without having to worry about eating. Overall, this meal plan can make your life easier.

When you can cut down on some of the work you need to do during the day and focus on something else, you may end up worrying about your life. We all know that stress can hurt our health and our lives. When you can reduce stress, it is easy to be the healthiest version of yourself.

Can Help with Cancer

Many people get cancer every year. This disease can lead to extreme conditions, and its characteristics include cells growing in an uncontrolled manner. Fasting is something that is said to be having great benefits in terms of your metabolism, which can lead to a reduction in cancer risk. Some human studies show that fasting cancer patients have been able to alleviate some of the chemical side effects.

Good on the Mind

Something considered to be working for the physical body could also work for the brain? Fasting can help improve the metabolic symptoms that are common in helping the brain stay healthy as well. This may include helping with insulin resistance, lowering blood sugar levels, reduced inflammation, and chemical stress.

There have been several studies conducted in rats showing how intermittent fasting can contribute to the growth of nerve cells, which improves brain function. Fasting can also help to increase the levels of brain activity that arise. When the brain is deficient in this, it can cause depression as well as other mental issues.

It Helps to Improve Cells

When we move fast, human cells can begin to be called the "resistance" of the digestive process. This involves breaking down the cells and metabolizing any proteins that are no longer used. As self-medication increases, it can help prevent human illnesses like cancer and Alzheimer's disease.

May Prevent Alzheimer's Disease

Alzheimer's is a neurological disease that has become common nowadays. The condition is not curable, and to ensure you are safe from it, prevention is better than cure. According to a particular study which was contacted on rats, one of the ways to prevent the disease is through intermittent fasting.

There are some cases whereby findings suggest that include fasting daily can have a positive impact when it comes to dealing with Alzheimer's disease. The studies have been done to both animals and human beings. Apart from this disease the studies also indicate that intermittent fasting can help in the prevention of other diseases like Parkinson's and Huntington diseases

Some case reports suggest that lifestyle changes (including daily or at least short-term fasting) help improve the symptoms of Alzheimer's disease in nine of the ten patients. Animal studies have also shown that this fasting can help prevent other neurological diseases such as Huntington's disease and Parkinson's disease.

Although most of these studies were done on animals, the results seemed promising. Temporary fasting is a trend, and research on its mechanisms for good health is not new. It takes time to learn all the benefits of fasting.

Regular Fasting Can Help You Live Longer

One of the most exciting things about interactive fasting is that it can help you live longer. Several studies in rodents have shown how intermittent fasting can help extend their lifespan—similar to what happens when you gradually reach the regular calorie limit. In some studies, the effect was surprisingly low. One is that animals that fast every day live 83% more than those that do not.

While it is difficult to justify an increase in its lifespan due to the intermittent fasting still has not been conducted in research on long-term populations to determine this, it is still a popular idea for those trying to prevent aging. Given the known benefits of the metabolism of this diet, it is no wonder that people believe that regular fasting will help them stay alive and healthy.

As you can see, there are many benefits to following a fast-food diet. We have only touched on a few of them, but there have been many studies on the effects of this diet and why it may be useful for you. If you are trying to improve your mental health, live longer, lose weight, or gain more energy, indirect fasting can improve your life.

Surviving Longer While Hungry

Hunger is feeling uncomfortable and/or being weak due to a lack of food. Hunger can be physical, but it can also just be a desire or want rather than a need right at that moment. The body sometimes responds as if its hunger, but sometimes we are thirsty and are yearning for liquids and not food; therefore, your water intake is imperative to your success in extending to longer fasting windows.

To habituate longer fasting windows and/or to resist food during your fasting window to make it to the feeding window, staying productive is vital. Stay busy by any means necessary. It is a great idea to exercise during this time or remain busy with your professional or personal work. Being lazy and feeling bored are false indicators to your body that you may be hungry when you are just in a slump or bored. The more you think about food, the weaker your body thinks your mind is, and eventually, this will be your takedown.

Chapter 3: Following the 16/8 Method Step-by-Step

We've already covered the basics of the 16/8 method, but here's a reminder. With the 16/8 method, you are fasting for 16 hours and eating within eight-hour. You'll have all your meals within these eight hours. Outside of them, have a lot of fluids (water, tea, black coffee) but no food and no sugar in your drinks. Remember, the 16/8 method is not a diet, just a specific time to eat.

Now that you know more about the fast, you may be ready just to jump right in and start! While this is an option, you might want to know more about what to do with the fast. In this chapter, we're going to cover what to do step-by-step. We're going to give you some guidance to transition into the 16/8 method. We'll also talk about what a month-long schedule might look like as you transition into the fast.

How to get started

We've talked a lot about the positives of the 16/8 method and how easy it is in comparison to other fasting methods. Please don't just jump into the fast. Immediately starting a fast without preparing your body can give you some dramatic hormone changes and mood changes. It can feel uncomfortable for the first couple of weeks before you start to feel better than before.

So, to reduce that discomfort, it's important to have a fasting plan and follow it. A fasting plan will include things like your goals, the times you're going to eat, what you're going to eat, and what signs might make you take a break from a fast. It's also where you can write down notes about how you're doing while fasting and areas where you can improve. A fasting plan will also help you restart your fast if you end up not fasting for a couple of weeks or months. The plan is a good reminder of how far you've come and what you can do to help you feel good on the fast. So, create a fasting plan. A lot of people like to keep this as a written journal, but you can also keep your notes in an app, on a spreadsheet, or your blog! Just make sure you have your plan and update it regularly. Once you have your notebook ready, here are our steps to transition into your fast.

Setting your goal

In your journal, write down your goals for fasting. Why do you want to follow the 16/8 method of fasting? Is it to be healthier, to manage medical issues, or just to feel better about your daily life? Have a specific reason for doing the 16/8 method. Having a goal can help keep you motivated to continue fasting, even during difficult times.

Your goal should be a SMART goal. SMART goals are goals that are specific, measurable, achievable, relevant and time-bound.

Specific. While you might say that your goal is to get healthier in general, this isn't a specific goal. A specific goal is clear and explains exactly where you want to see improvement. Do you want to have better blood sugar levels? Do you want to lose weight or inches from your waistline? Do you want to have more focus during your day? There are a variety of possible specific goals that you can choose from to start your fast.

Measurable. Your goal, whatever it is, should be measurable. There should be a measurement that helps you see that you've improved. Numbers are a great way to measure your goal's success, but it can also be something beyond numbers, like having a consistent mood. So long as you are tracking your goal and measuring it in some way, your goal will be measurable. If your goal is to have better blood sugar levels, then have a specific number you're aiming for every day. This number can be found by talking with your doctor. If your goal is to lose weight or inches, then have a specific number that you're looking for on the scale or the measuring tape. If your goal is to have more focus during the day, then track that feeling every day. Many people use mood trackers to help gauge their feelings every day. Trackers like this are perfect for non-tangible goals like feeling more focused, being happier, sleeping better, etc. When you can track your goals, then it is something measurable. If you aren't meeting your goals, you'll see that in your tracking, and you'll know that you need to adjust. And if you are meeting your goals, you can celebrate each milestone, and each moment you're closer to fully achieving your goal.

Achievable. Achievable goals are ones that you can reach. If your goal is to lose hundreds of pounds through fasting, that's not quite achievable or realistic. A better goal would be saying you want to lose ten pounds. This is an achievable goal. Once you meet this goal, feel free to create another one where you want to lose another ten pounds. Achievable goals should not be ones that are monumental or ones that are very idealistic. Choose realistic goals. We've talked before about how choosing a large goal is not likely to succeed. This is because large goals are often more like a vision far away rather than something that is smaller and doable. Having a large goal can cause your motivation to wane, which is why people often fail at New Year's resolutions. So, choose achievable goals. They don't have to be easy; they just must be possible.

Relevant. Let's say that you and your best friend B decide to do the 16/8 method together. This is honestly great because you'll have someone you're accountable to and someone who supports you. But your goals for the fast should not be the same. Your goals need to be relevant to you. Hugh Jackman did the 16/8 method for preparing his Wolverine role. Does this mean that you should follow his same goals of muscle growth and weight loss? No. He had trainers, nutritionists, and coaches that helped him reach those goals. You probably don't have that support. Besides, are you trying to look like Wolverine? Probably not. Choose goals that are relevant to you personally. Choose the measurements that work for you. Friend B might want to lose 20 pounds, but you might want just to sleep better. So long as the goal is yours, it will be relevant.

Time-bound. Goals that have a specific time to be achieved are beneficial. This doesn't mean that once you've reached your goal, you stop. You can stop if you want to, but you can also repeat the same goal or make another goal to follow. If your goal is to have better blood sugar levels, when do you want this to happen? If you want to lose weight, when will you achieve this goal? If you want to have more focus at work, at what point will you say you've achieved your goals?

Planning Your sleeping and eating Schedule

This is a critical step. You can plan what to eat and where to eat it, but with the 16/8 method, it's all about when you eat. Remember, you only have an eight-hour window to eat, so what time will you have breakfast (or will you not have breakfast), what time will you have lunch, and when will you have dinner? Consider things like your current work schedule or family schedule. Do you want to eat dinner right before the beginning of your fasting time, or do you want to eat it a bit earlier? Consider all these factors. If you exercise regularly, you'll want to eat immediately after eating. However, this is just a suggestion. Some people feel weak if they don't eat something before exercising, so choose your schedule based on your feeling. Also, consider special events. How will your schedule change have based on these events? At the end of this chapter, we'll share some example fasting schedules, but be sure to adapt them to your own life.

During your day, your metabolism is often fastest in the morning and slumps around 3:00 p.m. At this point, it begins its slow-down process preparing for the night. So, you can choose to have your eating window from 7:00 a.m. to 3:00 p.m. and eat your meals there, following your circadian rhythm. However, remember that this schedule doesn't work for everyone. It also doesn't give you the opportunity to eat during social events in the evening. While it doesn't give you a social life mealtime, you can always adjust your fasting and eating window to fit a planned event. You don't want to be the only one at the table which is drinking a glass of water while everyone else eats. So, plan when you'll eat to fit your lifestyle.

It's ideal to follow the 16/8 method daily, and most people do. However, you don't have to! Some people follow it during the workweek but then skip the weekends to better fit in social eating and drinking. Choose whatever will work for you. You can also work with your doctor to help plan out your schedule.

While we're talking about schedules, it's also important to have a consistent sleep schedule. Set a consistent time to go to bed and a consistent time to wake up and follow it. This will help you figure out how many hours you need to fast each day. If you're going to go to bed at 11:00 p.m. and wake up at 7: a.m., then you can fit your fasting schedule around that. You could do your additional eight hours of fasting before you go to bed, or you could divide it into four hours before bed and four hours after you wake up. If you have a consistent sleep time but don't follow it, then it's useless. So, make sure you're following it. If you know it takes you 30 minutes of downtime before you fall asleep, then be in bed 30 minutes earlier, read a book, have some water, and then try to fall asleep at your set time. Use your alarm clock to wake up and don't keep hitting the snooze button. Overall, this consistency will help you better manage your fast.

What to drink

Here comes the science. You need to find meals that will fit in your daily nutrition requirements and calories and keep you full. Consider snacks. Will you snack during your day? How will you break your fast? With a full meal, protein drink, or nothing? All of this should take into consideration your daily activities. If you're exercising, you'll want to make sure you have enough energy to exercise and not be hungry during the fasting period. You can experiment with meals and then write down the results of those meals in your fasting journal. Did you feel hungry quickly after eating? Then you'll need to change your meal. If you find that you're craving something, then you might be missing a nutrient in your meal. For example, if you're craving peanut butter, add more protein to your meals. In general, the health department has some good guidelines for how many calories to eat per day. You can then divide these calories into your meals and your snacks (if you choose to snack). All this information below is from health.gov. Because these values are for an "average" adult in height and weight, you'll need to calculate it further based on your weight and height. You can use various websites to find the right calories for maintaining or losing weight.

Keeping a progress journal

This isn't really a requirement, but many people find it incredibly motivating. Not only can it motivate you, but you're before the picture can motivate others too. If you look at a variety of blogs about people's journeys with fasting, you'll always see a before and after/current picture. This can be really motivating for the person in the picture to see their change. Seeing the physical differences in your body from before and after your fast can make you feel happy. So, take a before picture! Add it to your journal, and as you reach some of your goals, take other pictures to commemorate your success.

Sleeping Well the Night before You Start

Now we're getting into starting the fast. The day before you start your new fast, you want to make sure you begin your preparation. Try to sleep well before you start. This will help your body prepare itself and start the process of syncing your circadian rhythm. Remember, it's a process, and you want to start on the right foot. The next day (day 1 of your fast), have a good breakfast. That night, you'll start your fasting hours.

How to exercise safely during the 16/8 fast

Start your fast gradually. Don't start by doing all 16 hours at once. Instead, break it down over the course of a couple of weeks. Assuming you sleep for eight hours a night, you only need to fast an additional eight hours during your waking hours. In week 1, for the first three days, stop eating an hour before you go to bed, and start eating one hour after you wake up. This puts you at a 10-hour fast, with 14 hours to eat. After those first three days, you're going to add an hour to before bed and after waking up. So, you'll stop eating two hours before bed and start eating two hours after waking up. This puts you at a 12-hour fast, with 12 hours to eat. Three days later, add another two hours, bringing you up to a 14-hour fast, and a 10-hour eating period. Then finally, extend to the full 16 hours of fasting and 8 hours of eating. This should slowly get you into the full fast and help curb the discomfort you might feel. This will take about two weeks to get to the full fast.

One thing to mention is that exercise should be reduced during this time, and water consumption should be increased. As you get used to the fast, you can increase your exercise, but just at the beginning, you might struggle with exercising with fasting. You should also be drinking a lot more liquid as you transition into the fast. You'll want to keep hydrated because your body will start noticing that there is a larger and larger window of nothing coming in. Have water to keep you hydrated and help curb your appetite if you're feeling hungry during your fasting window.

You are, of course, welcome to just jump in and do the full 16 hours of fasting and 8 hours of eating, but with this jump into fasting, you'll have some discomfort for the first week or so. We'll discuss discomfort in the next step.

How to deal with Discomfort

While starting your fast, you need to prepare yourself for some changes to your body and habits. You might feel some discomfort with the change. This includes things like strange sleep patterns or dreams, changes in your mood, and sometimes bloating or digestive discomfort. These will usually pass after a couple of weeks of fasting. Some people are lucky and never feel discomfort, but others do. Take the time to evaluate what you're feeling. If something is feeling way off, stop fasting, and talk to your doctor. Signs that you have to stop and talk with your doctor are feelings of weakness and dizziness, changes to your heart rate or respiration, and severe discomfort.

Likely, you'll also feel some positive changes within the first week. Many people feel like their brains are clearer. This means that they have more focus and awareness of their environment, with less fogginess. This is a great feeling. It comes with the changes to your hormonal patterns but also the reset to your circadian rhythm. Embrace the change! Within a couple of weeks, you'll notice other changes. In research, after eight weeks of fasting, there were decent metabolic changes that people were able to maintain. This includes changes to blood glucose levels, insulin levels, and other hormones. These changes will make you feel better than you're used to, which is a great benefit that comes with fasting.

How to stay motivated

The final step is to keep track of your progress and record it all in your fasting journal. Note times when your meals didn't work out and times when they did. Also, record times when you felt discomfort and times when you felt fantastic with your fast! Include pictures, little motivational notes—really, anything that will help you keep on track.

Check your journal regularly. This can give you some motivation, but it can also help you find areas to tweak your fast to better fit in your life. Your journal is your journey recorded. You can use it to help motivate others but also remind you of the progress you have made. Keep it up and keep recording your progress.

PART TWO: MEAL PLAN AND RECIPES

Chapter 4: Sample Meal Plan for 16/8 IF

DAYS	BREAKFAST	LUNCH/DINNER	SNACK/DESSERT
1	Choco Chip Whey Waffles	Spicy Pork Chops	Lemon Broccoli
2	Coco Cinnamon-Packed Pancakes	Paprika Lamb Chops	Philadelphia Potato Praline
3	Magdalena Muffins with Tart Tomatoes	Delicious Turkey Wrap	Stuffed Mushrooms
4	Spinach Shoots Mediterranean Medley	Creamy Kale and Mushrooms	Parmesan Crisps
5	Romantic Raspberry Power Pancake	Cauliflower Fritters	Coconut Peanut Butter Fudge
6	Spinach Sausage Feta Frittata	Grilled Parmesan Eggplant	Raspberry Chia Pudding
7	Mayonnaise Mixed with Energy Egg	Creamy Artichoke and Spinach	Chocó Chia Pudding

Chapter 5: Foods to Enjoy/Avoid on 16:8

What to eat while fasting and what not to eat

While there are no specific food guidelines as to how you should make up the "Eating" portions of the day, we recommend that you try to stay away from processed food as much as possible and stick to natural alternatives.

Healthy Fats: It is really good for you to consume healthy fats when staying in a clean eating diet. Go for the following

- Olive oil
- Extra Virgin Olive Oil
- Organic Unsalted Butter
- Coconut Oil
- Organic Ghee
- Sunflower Oil

- Avocado

Flours and Grains: Always make sure that you are using 100% whole grain flours that have no additives or preservatives.

- Bread
- Pasta
- Tortillas
- Rice
- Flours

- Soba Noodles
- Cornmeal
- Bread Crumbs

Dairy: Always go for full-fat organic and grass-fed dairy products.

- Plain yogurt
- Buttermilk
- Greek Yogurt
- Sour Cream
- Cream Cheese
- Cottage Cheese
- Milk
- Cheese

Nondairy/Protein Alternative: For protein alternatives, it is good to go for unsweetened plain almond, soy sauce, coconut milk, or even rice.

- Organic Tofu
- Organic Tempeh

Seafood: Sustainable shellfish and fish are the best choices when considering seafood.

Produce: Organic products such as vegetables and fruits are always great for a clean diet.

Meats: When going for meat, it is essential that you go for hormone and antibiotic-free organic meats.

- Poultry
- All-natural bacon
- Uncured deli meats such as ham
- Lean red meats

Salts and Herb: Salts and herbs are self-explanatory. Use them in reasonable amounts.

- Herbs
- Kosher salt or sea salt

Nuts: Nuts as seeds are allowed in a clean diet, so use them liberally

- Unsalted nuts and seeds
- Organic unsalted seed butter/ nut butter

Sweeteners: It is essential that you keep your sugar intake to an as low level as possible, but if your sweet tooth is tingling too much! Then simply go for the following CE approved sweeteners.

- Raw honey
- Date sugar
- Pure maple syrup
- Stevia
- Organic Evaporated cane juice
- Dark chocolate

- Pure vanilla extract

- Unsweetened shredded coconut

Juices: Always go for 100% pure juices!

- Lemon juice (100%)

- 100% fruit juice

- Cold-pressed or homemade 100% vegetable and fruit juices

Thickeners: Some thickeners are allowed in a clean diet such as

- Arrowroot

- Tapioca Starch

- Potato Starch

Canned and Jarred Produce: For canned goods such as tomatoes or beans, only go for the ones that are BPA free.

Condiments: One thing to note while purchasing condiments is to look for the labels. Make sure that they contain no additives, preservatives, or sugar. Alternatively, if possible, then try to make your own.

- Hot Sauce

- Dijon Mustard

- Reduced Sodium Soy Sauce

- Vinegar

Some additional ingredients: Some more that you should know about:

- Dried berries that are unsweetened
- Liquid smoke naturally crafted
- The chicken broth that is low in sodium
- Agar
- Tomato paste (unsalted)

How to identify processed food

The quick pointers below will help you to a clearer idea of how you can identify processed foods.

☐ Foods that contain any kind of preservatives such as salt, flavor, or sugar to extend their shelf life are processed food. This includes beverages as well as breakfast cereals.

☐ Any kind of food that has its natural form altered should be considered as processed food. For example, bread with their bran and germ removed are to be considered as processed food.

☐ Foods that contain one or more artificially created components are considered as processed food.

How should you calculate your calorie intake?

This is something that you should pay very close attention to as having a proper calorie intake/burn rate is crucial to how much weight you will lose in the long run.

You may have noticed while browsing through various food labels that the given values are specified to be "Percent of daily values". Now, you might be curious to know what does that exactly means.

Well, it means that those particular nutritional values are presented and calculated considering a scenario where an average person eats 2000 calories in one day. But this is not made in stones as the physiology and requirements of every single human being varies from one to the next, and your daily intake might be greater than 2000 calories.

Other factors that come into consideration are height, age, weight, gender, and level of daily physical activity.

Now, before you set up your weight loss target, it is important that you know how should calculate your daily calorie intake.

While calculating your daily calorie intake, there are certain factors that you are to consider and keep in mind, such as:

- Thermic effect of food
- Physical activity
- Basal activity

And as for the actual procedure, we need to talk about something known as "BMR".

Just in case you don't know, the Basal Metabolic Rate is the minimum level of calories required by your body to keep it healthy in a resting state.

This particular value amounts to almost 60-70% of the calories that you burn each day. Keep in mind that generally speaking, men have a much higher BMR than women.

While there are many ways of calculating this, the most prominent method of calculating the basal metabolic rate is through the usage of the "Harris Benedict" method, which is illustrated below:

Once you have figured out your BMR, the next step would you to calculate your total calorie requirements.

To do that, just simply follow the given steps based on your level of activity

- If you have almost no physical activity, then calculating your calorie intake is as simple as = BMR value x 1.2
- If you have the tendency to do light exercise and/or workout around 1-3 days per week, then your calorie calculation would be = BMR value x 1.375
- If you tend to do moderate levels of workout, around 3-5 days per week, then your calorie intake would be = BMR x 1.55
- If you have the tendency to do high levels of exercise, mainly around 6-7 days per week, then your calorie intake would be calculated by = BMR x 1.55

- And lastly, if you do very hard physical exercise/ sports activity, then your calorie intake should be calculated using= BMR x 1.9

Let me give you an example to makes it clearer.

So, let's consider that you are sedentary and have low levels of physical activity.

You calculate and find out that your BMR is 1745

So, multiplying it by 1.2, you would get 2094, which is the total amount of calories that you need daily to maintain the current weight level of yours.

Calorie for losing weight

Now that the basic concepts of calorie intake are cleared up, the next step for you is to understand how you can actually start to lose weight while with that knowledge.

So, the first thing that you must understand is that there are approximately 3500 calories in a pound of your stored body fat. So, if you want to lose body fat, what you have to do essentially is burn 3500 calories either through dieting or physical exercise, or using both of them combined.

If you can create a calorie gap of 7000, then you will be able to burn 2 pounds in a week. The amount of stress that your body is able to take will ultimately depend on your will power and stress levels.

The calorie deficit can be brought upon by either eating less or eating low-calorie food/having more physical activity.

 The most preferred way is to have a combination of a healthy diet and a good amount of physical activity in order to get the best out of it.

If you want to lose your weight, the general guideline that you should follow is to lower your calorie intake by at least 500, but making sure that you don't cross 1000 at it might hamper your normal activities.

On the other hand, if you want to lose just a small amount, then 1000 calories might be too much, so go for lower deficit targets.

As recommended by the American College of Sports Medicine or ACSM, your calorie intake should never drop below 1200 per day if you are a female and 1800 if you are a female.

Next, we will talk about how Intermittent Fasting affects the hormones of your body. But before that, let me clear up what "Hormones" actually are.

Chapter 6: Intermittent Fasting Recipes

Breakfast Ideas

Choco Chip Whey Waffles

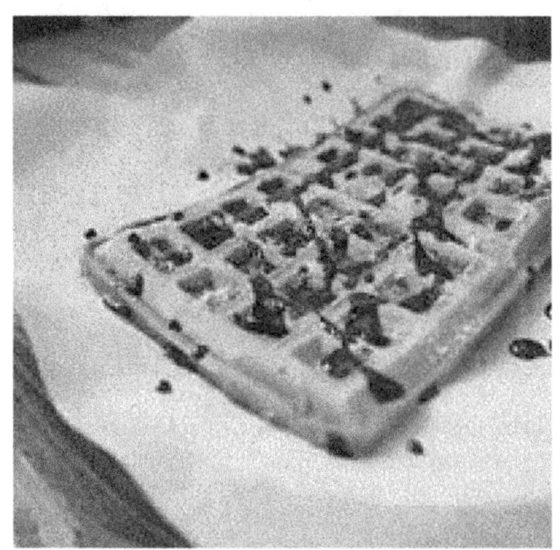

Servings: 2

Preparation time 10 minutes

Cooking Time: 6 minutes

Ingredients:

2-tbsp organic coconut oil

2-tbsp coconut sugar

4-tbsp chocolate whey protein powder

⅓-cup almond flour

A pinch of salt

½-tsp baking powder

½-cup almond milk

2-pcs eggs

Directions:

Mix all the ingredients in the blender to obtain a homogenous paste.

Preheat your waffle iron. Pour the waffle dough in the iron and cook each waffle for 3 minutes.

Nutrition:

Calories: 423

Fat: 32.8g Protein: 26.5g Total Carbohydrates: 8.3g Dietary Fiber: 2.9g Net Carbohydrates: 5.4g

Coco Cinnamon-Packed Pancakes

Servings: 2

Preparation time 30 minutes

Cooking Time: 5 minutes

Ingredients:

2-pcs eggs

2½-tbsp organic coconut flour

¼-cup milk substitute with hydrogenated vegetable oil (or almond milk)

1-tbsp baking soda

½-tbsp cinnamon

½-tbsp baobab powder

2-tbsp organic coconut flower syrup

Directions:

In a salad bowl, mix the coconut flour, baobab powder, cinnamon, and baking soda.

Add the beaten eggs, the almond milk, and the coconut syrup. Let the dough rest for 30 minutes.

Cook the pancakes in a hot pan with coconut oil.

Dress the pancakes with raspberries/blueberries or almonds.

Nutrition:

Calories: 392

Fat: 32.5g Protein: 20g Total Carbohydrates: 11.3g Dietary Fiber: 6.4g Net Carbohydrates: 4.9g

Magdalena Muffins with Tart Tomatoes

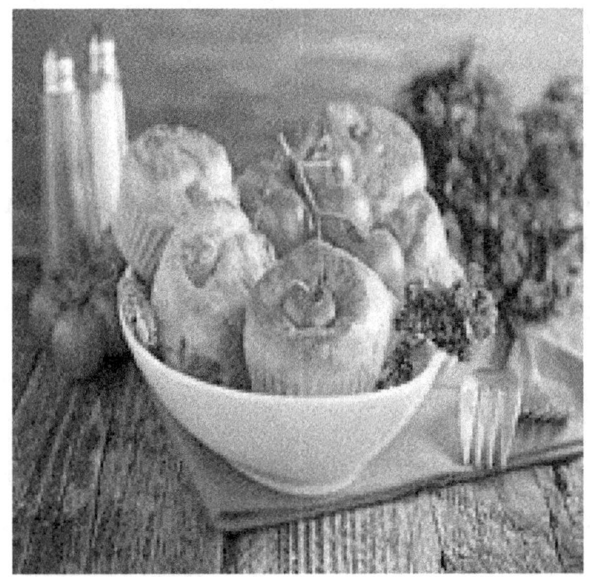

Servings: 2

Preparation time 10 minutes

Cooking Time: 20 minutes

Ingredients:

2½-tbsp whole-wheat flour

2½-tbsp almond flour

1-tbsp yeast or baking soda

A dash of salt, pepper, and paprika

2-pcs eggs

1-tbsp organic cashew nuts

1-tbsp hemp oil

2½-tbsp soymilk

⅓-cup feta cheese, diced

1⅓-cup dried tomatoes, without oil and sliced into small pieces

Directions:

Mix the wheat flour, almond flour, yeast, and spices.

Then add eggs, cashews, oil, and soymilk.

Mix well to obtain a smooth paste. Add the feta and tomatoes.

Mix well and pour the dough into muffin pans previously greased with coconut oil.

Bake for 20 minutes at 350°F.

Nutrition:

Calories: 405

Fat: 33.3g Protein: 20.3g Total Carbohydrates: 11g Dietary Fiber: 4.9g Net Carbohydrates: 6.1g

Spinach Shoots Mediterranean Medley

Servings: 2

Preparation time 10 minutes

Cooking Time: 1 minute

Ingredients:

½-cup spinach shoots

2-tbsp quinoa

¼-cup avocado, sliced

1-tbsp fresh goat cheese

1-tsp agave syrup, gluten-free

¼-cup dried blackberries

1-pc fig

1-tsp pumpkin seeds puree

Directions:

Arrange the spinach shoots, cooked quinoa, and avocado on a large plate.

Mix the goat cheese, agave syrup, and dried blackberries.

Make 4 small cuts in the fig so that you can open it and insert the goat cheese mixture.

Spread your fig on the spinach shoots. Sprinkle over with pumpkin seed puree.

Nutrition:

Calories: 308

Fat: 26g Protein: 15.4g Total Carbohydrates: 9.7g Dietary Fiber: 6.5g Net Carbohydrates: 3.2g

Romantic Raspberry Power Pancake

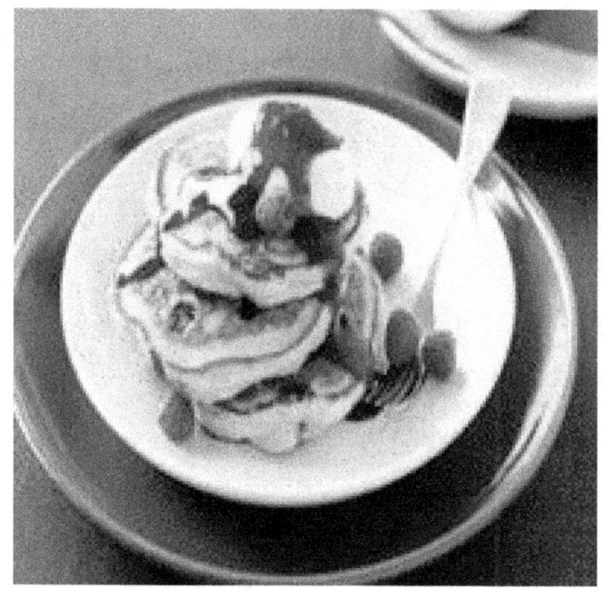

Serving: 1

Preparation time 5 minutes

Cooking Time: 10 minutes

Ingredients:

2-tbsp raspberries, crushed

2-tsp almond flour

1-tbsp yeast or baking soda

1-tbsp vegan protein powder

2-tbsp soymilk

1-tbsp coconut oil

Directions:

Mix the crushed raspberries and dry ingredients.

Pour the milk and mix well to obtain a homogenous mixture.

Cook the pancakes for 2 minutes on each side using a little coconut oil in a pan. Flip the pancake when small bubbles appear.

Dress with almonds or nuts.

Nutrition:

Calories: 323

Fat: 25.3g Protein: 15.7g Total Carbohydrates: 12g Dietary Fiber: 3.8g Net Carbohydrates: 4.8g

Spinach Sausage Feta Frittata

Servings: 6

Preparation time 15 minutes

Cooking Time: 30 minutes

Ingredients:

10-oz. spinach, frozen, thawed, drained, and chopped

12-oz. sausage, sliced into small pieces

½-cup feta cheese, crumbled

½-cup almond milk, unsweetened

½-cup heavy cream

¼-tsp. ground nutmeg

½-tsp. salt

¼-tsp. black pepper

12-pcs eggs whisked

Directions:

Place the sausage in a medium-sized mixing bowl. Break the spinach up into the same bowl as the sausage.

Sprinkle the cheese over the mixture. Toss lightly until fully combined. Lightly spread the mixture onto a greased 13" × 9" casserole dish or greased muffin cups.

In a larger bowl, blend the almond milk, cream, nutmeg, salt, and pepper with the eggs, and mix well until fully combined.

Gently pour the mixture into the dish or muffin cups until for about ¾ full. Bake at 375°F for about 50 minutes (for the casserole), or 30 minutes (for the muffin cups), or until fully set.

Nutrition:

Calories: 295

Fat: 22.9g Protein: 18.5g Total Carbohydrates: 4.6g Dietary Fiber: 1g Net Carbohydrates: 3.6g

Mayonnaise Mixed with Energy Egg

Serving: 1

Preparation time 2 minutes

Cooking Time: 5 minutes

Ingredients:

2-tbsp organic mayonnaise, gluten-free

1-pc large egg

1-tbsp butter

Directions:

Mix the mayonnaise and egg in a medium-sized bowl until fully combined.

Melt the butter in a non-stick skillet. Pour the egg mixture, and cook until set. Scrape the egg and all remaining fat onto a serving plate. Serve immediately.

Nutrition:

Calories: 295

Fat: 22.7g Protein: 18.8g Total Carbohydrates: 3.8g Dietary Fiber: 0.1g Net Carbohydrates: 3.7g

Avocados atop Toasted Tartiné

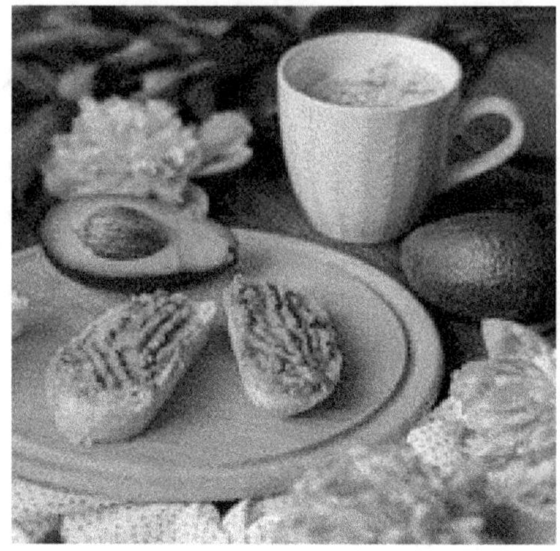

Servings: 2

Preparation time 10 minutes

Cooking Time: 5 minutes

Ingredients:

2-slices bread, gluten-free

½-pc small avocado, thinly sliced

1-tbsp fresh cheese

1-tsp lemon juice

A dash of salt and pepper

1-tsp chia seeds for garnish (optional)

Directions:

Toast the bread slices lightly.

Carefully arrange the avocado slices on each bread slice. Drizzle with the lemon juice. Spread the fresh cheese. Sprinkle with pepper and salt. Top with garnish.

Nutrition:

Calories: 268

Fat: 22.4g Protein: 13.5g Total Carbohydrates: 8.9g Dietary Fiber: 6.7g Net Carbohydrates: 3.2g

Fish Fillet & Perky Potato Cheese Combo

Servings: 2

Preparation time 15 minutes

Cooking Time: 10 minutes

Ingredients:

1-tbsp olive oil

1-pc large potato, cooked and thinly sliced

¼-cup lean white cheese

½-tsp herbs of your choice

3.5-oz. herring fillet, steamed and sliced in half

½-tsp flaxseed oil or coconut oil

A dash of salt and pepper

Directions:

Heat a non-stick pan with olive oil. Add potato slices and cook for several minutes until browned.

Season the white cheese with salt, pepper, and herbs of your choice.

Arrange the potatoes equally between two plates. Top with the cheese and herring fillets. Garnish with a drizzle of flaxseed oil.

Nutrition:

Calories: 298

Fat: 24.9g Protein: 14.2g Total Carbohydrates: 6.5g Dietary Fiber: 3.2g Net Carbohydrates: 4.3g

Cream Cheese Protein Pancake

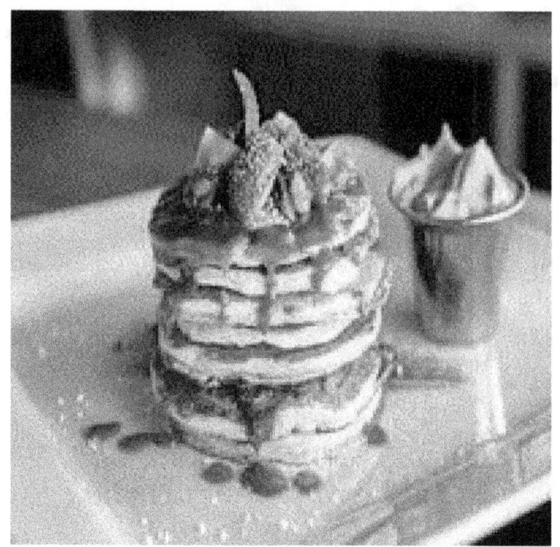

Servings: 2

Preparation time 10 minutes

Cooking Time: 12 minutes

Ingredients:

2-pcs eggs

2-oz cream cheese

1-packet sweetener

½-tsp cinnamon

1-tbsp butter

Directions:

Mix all the ingredients in a blender except the butter. Blend until smooth. Let the batter stand for 2 minutes to allow the bubbles to settle.

Grease slightly a hot pan with ¼-tbsp butter. Pour ¼-batter into the pan. Cook for about 2 minutes until turning golden. Flip the pancake and cook for 1 minute on its other side.

Repeat the same cooking procedure with the remaining batter. Serve with fresh berries of choice and sugar-free syrup.

Nutrition:

Calories: 340

Fat: 28.1g Protein: 16.2g Total Carbohydrates: 8.1g Dietary Fiber: 3.8g Net Carbohydrates: 4.3g

Veggie Variety with Peanut Paste

Serving: 1

Preparation time 15 minutes

Cooking Time: 15 minutes

Ingredients:

1-bulb small onion, thinly sliced

¾-cup broccoli, sliced into quarters

1-pc small carrot, sliced into quarters

½-pc green pepper, thinly sliced

5-pcs mushrooms, sliced into quarters

A dash of salt, pepper, and powdered chili

2-tbsp peanut butter, dairy-free

2-tbsp. soy sauce, gluten-free

1-tbsp agave syrup (or honey), gluten-free

¼-cup red cabbage, thinly sliced

Directions:

Pour a little water in a heated skillet and cook the onions until they are transparent. Add the broccoli, carrot, pepper, and mushrooms. Cook for 10 minutes until tender. (Add some water if the pan is too dry). Season the veggies with a dash of salt, pepper, and chili.

For the sauce, mix the peanut butter with the soy sauce, agave syrup, and 3 tbsp water.

To serve, incorporate the red cabbage. Garnish the dish with the sauce.

Nutrition:

Calories: 349

Fat: 28.7g Protein: 18.4g Total Carbohydrates: 10.8g Dietary Fiber: 6.5g Net Carbohydrates: 4.3g

Avocado Aliment with Egg Element

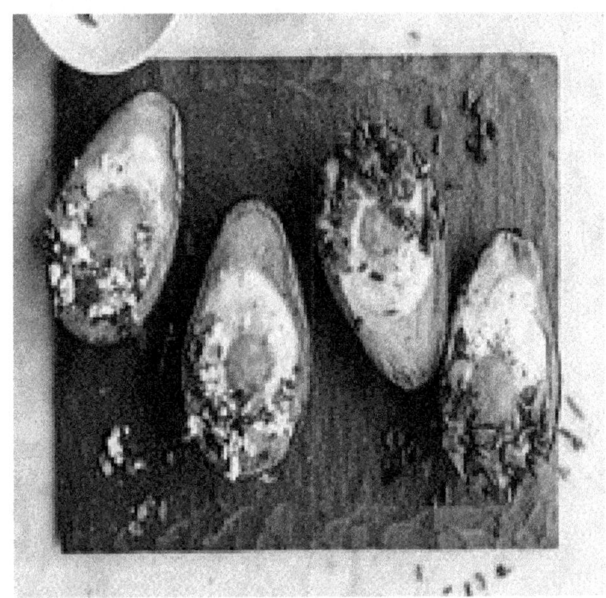

Servings: 2

Preparation time 8 minutes

Cooking Time: 20 minutes

Ingredients:

1 egg, whisked

1 avocado, halved, pitted, and removed slightly with flesh

A dash of sea salt and pepper

1-tbsp parsley, chopped

1-tsp cayenne pepper

Directions:

Preheat your oven to 375°F.

Pour the egg gently into each halved avocado. Remove the excess liquid.

Place the stuffed avocado in a baking tray. Bake for 20 minutes.

Season the preparation with sea salt, parsley, and cayenne pepper.

Nutrition:

Calories: 275

Fat: 23.8g Protein: 11.8g Total Carbohydrates: 10.7g Dietary Fiber: 4g Net Carbohydrates: 3.4g

Pumpkin Pancakes

Servings: 3

Preparation time 10 minutes

Cooking Time: 30 minutes

Ingredients:

1-tsp vanilla extract

1-cup coconut cream

3-pcs eggs

2-tbsp egg whites

½-cup pumpkin puree

5-packs sweetener

4-tbsp ground flax seed

4-tbsp ground hazelnuts or hazelnut flour

1-tsp yeast or baking powder

1-tbsp black tea powder

1-tbsp. coconut oil for cooking

Directions:

Whisk together the first five liquid ingredients for half a minute until they become frothy. Mix the dry ingredients in a separate bowl.

Combine both the dry and liquid ingredients to obtain a batter. (Add water, as necessary if the mixture is too thick.)

Grease a saucepan with a teaspoon of coconut oil. Ladle in the first pancake.

Cover the pan and cook for 3 minutes. Flip and cook the other side.

Repeat the cooking process until using up all the batter.

Nutrition:

Calories: 200

Fat: 16.4g Protein: 11g Total Carbohydrates: 5.2g Dietary Fiber: 3g Net Carbohydrates: 2.2g

Whole-Wheat Plain Pancakes

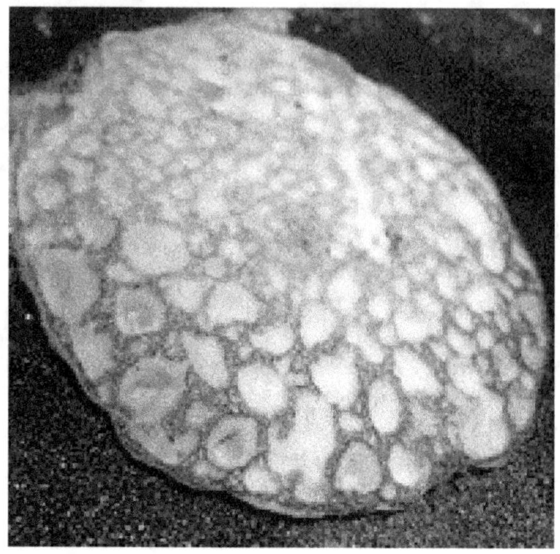

Serving: 1

Preparation time 5 minutes

Cooking Time: 12 minutes

Ingredients:

2-pcs eggs

4-tbsp whole-wheat flour

½-tsp yeast or baking soda

⅓-cup sunflower oil

1-tbsp coconut oil for cooking

Directions:

Mix all the ingredients in a bowl until obtaining a smooth consistency.

Pour the coconut oil in a pan placed over medium heat. Cook for 3 minutes until browned. Flip and cook the other side.

Serve hot and garnish with fresh fruits of your choice such as blueberries, strawberries or raspberries, nuts, and coconut flakes.

Nutrition:

Calories: 329

Fat: 27.6g Protein: 16.1g Total Carbohydrates: 5.4g Dietary Fiber: 1.3g Net Carbohydrates: 4.4g

Blueberries Breakfast Bowl

Serving: 1

Preparation time 35 minutes

Cooking Time: 0 minutes

Ingredients:

1-tsp chia seeds

1-cup almond milk

¼-cup fresh blueberries or fresh fruits

1-pack sweetener for taste

Directions:

Mix the chia seeds with almond milk. Stir periodically.

Place in the fridge to cool for 30 minutes, and then serve with fresh fruit. Enjoy!

Nutrition:

Calories: 202

Fat: 16.8g Protein: 10.2g Total Carbohydrates: 9.8g Dietary Fiber: 5.8g Net Carbohydrates: 2.6g

Feta-Filled Tomato-Topped Oldie Omelet

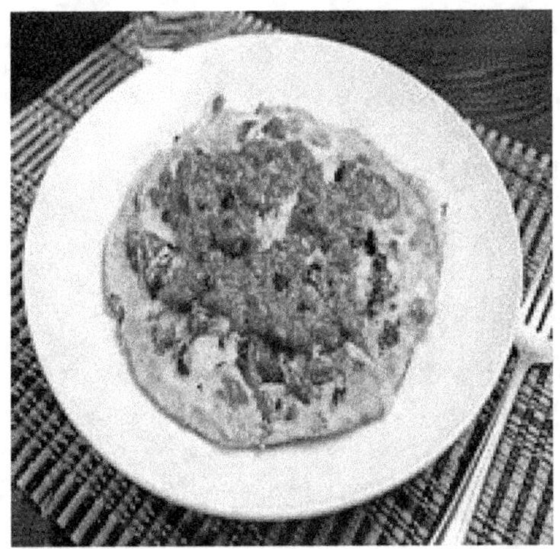

Serving: 1

Preparation time 5 minutes

Cooking Time: 6 minutes

Ingredients:

1-tbsp coconut oil

2-pcs eggs

1½-tbsp milk

A dash of salt and pepper

¼-cup tomatoes, sliced into cubes

2-tbsp feta cheese, crumbled

Directions:

Beat the eggs with the pepper, salt, milk, and the remaining spices.

Pour the mixture into a heated pan with coconut oil.

Stir in the tomatoes and cheese. Cook for 6 minutes or until the cheese melts.

Nutrition:

Calories: 335

Fat: 28.4g Protein: 16.2g Total Carbohydrates: 4.5g Dietary Fiber: 0.8g Net Carbohydrates: 3.7g

Ave Avocado Super Smoothie

Serving: 1

Preparation time 10 minutes

Cooking Time: 1 minute

Ingredients:

½-cup Greek yogurt

7-oz. frozen avocados

½-cup water

½-tsp vanilla powder

1-tsp each chia seeds, chocolate chips, and peanut butter for garnish

Directions:

Mix all the ingredients. You can also use a blender to crush them.

Pour the smoothie into a bowl and garnish to your taste with fruits, seeds, or nuts.

Nutrition:

Calories: 398

Fat: 33.1g Protein: 20g Total Carbohydrates: 15.5g Dietary Fiber: 10.6g Net Carbohydrates: 4.9g

Hearty Hodgepodge

Serving: 1

Preparation time 5 minutes

Cooking Time: 25 minutes

Ingredients:

1-bulb small onion, diced

1-tbsp coconut oil

1-tbsp bacon bits

1-pc medium zucchini, diced into squares

1-tbsp parsley or chives, chopped

¼-tsp. of salt

1-pc large egg, fried

Directions:

Sauté the onion with coconut oil in a pan placed over medium heat. Add the bacon, frequently stirring until both onion and bacon turn slightly brown.

Add the zucchini, and cook for 15 minutes. Remove from heat and transfer the preparation in a serving bowl. Sprinkle over the parsley.

To serve, top the dish with the fried egg.

Nutrition:

Calories: 290

Fat: 24g Protein: 14.6g Total Carbohydrates: 6.7g Dietary Fiber: 3.1g Net Carbohydrates: 3.6g

Chocolate Chia Plain Pudding

Servings: 3

Preparation time 55 minutes

Cooking Time: 0 minutes

Ingredients:

3-tbsp chia seeds

2-cups water

¼-cup whey chocolate protein

½-cup Greek yogurt, sugar-free

¼-cup linseeds, roasted

1-tbsp cocoa powder, unsweetened

1-packet sweetener (optional)

Directions:

Add chia seeds to a bowl of water and let stand for 20 minutes while occasionally stirring.

When chia seeds are inflated, add the other ingredients, and mix again.

Refrigerate for 30 minutes before serving.

Nutrition:

Calories: 370

Fat: 28.7g Protein: 22.3g Total Carbohydrates: 10.8g Dietary Fiber: 5.2g Net Carbohydrates: 5.6g

Seasoned Sardines with Sunny Side

Serving: 1

Preparation time 5 minutes

Cooking Time: 10 minutes

Ingredients:

2-oz. sardines in olive oil

2-pcs eggs

½-cup arugula

¼-cup artichoke hearts, diced

A pinch of salt

A dash of black pepper

Directions:

Preheat your oven to 375°F.

Place the sardines in an oven-ready stoneware bowl. Add the eggs on top of the sardines. Top the eggs with the arugula and artichokes. Sprinkle with salt and pepper.

Bake for 10 minutes until the eggs cook through.

Nutrition:

Calories: 255

Fat: 21g Protein: 13.5g Total Carbohydrates: 4.9g Dietary Fiber: 1.8g Net Carbohydrates: 3.1g

Healthy Breakfast Burritos

Servings: 4

Prep time - 5 mins Cooking time - 10 mins

Ingredients

8 eggs

1 tbsp milk

1 tbsp garlic, minced

1 red pepper, minced

Half an onion, red if possible, minced

4 slices of bacon, cooked

Salt

Pepper

4 tortilla wraps (multi-grain or wholegrain)

little cheese (optional)

Directions:

Take a medium-sized saucepan and heat over a medium heat

Add the garlic and cook for a couple of minutes, until fragrant

Whisk the eggs with the milk and place to one side

Add the pepper and onion to the pan and allow to cook for a couple more minutes

Add the eggs to the pan and cook for 4 minutes

Once cooked, add a quarter of the egg mixture onto each tortilla wrap and add one piece of the bacon on top

You can add cheese if you want, although it isn't necessary

Wrap up and enjoy it!

Nutrition:

Calories: 352

Carbs: 22g Fat: 20g Protein: 8g

Lunch Ideas

Mongolian Beef

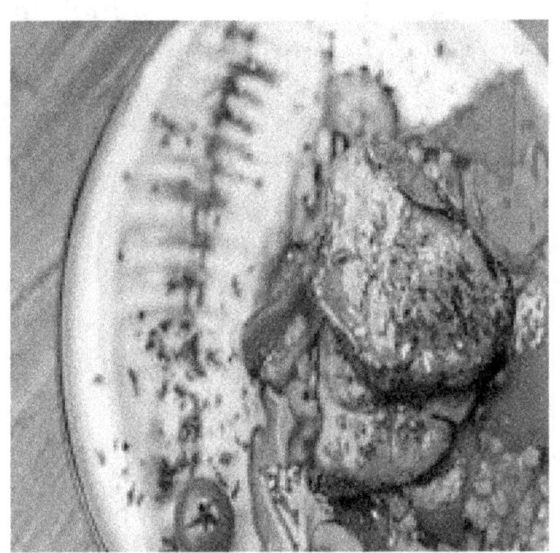

Servings: 4

Preparation time 10 minutes

Cooking time: 20

Ingredients

2 teaspoons Asian garlic chili paste

2 teaspoons vegetable oil

1 tablespoon rice vinegar

1 pound sirloin beef, lean and cubed

16 green onions, chopped

1 tablespoon ginger minced

2 tablespoons low soy sauce

1 garlic clove, minced

1 teaspoon cornstarch

1 tablespoon hoisin sauce

Directions

Take a bowl and stir in soy sauce, cornstarch, hoisin sauce, rice vinegar, chili paste

Add ginger, garlic, beef to a heated skillet and Sauté for 3 minutes until the beef is nice and golden

Mix in sauce, green onions and cook for a few minutes

Enjoy!

Nutrition Values (Per Serving)

Calorie: 231

Fat: 7g

Carbohydrates: 10g

Protein: 27g

Western Pork Chops

Servings: 4

Preparation time 10 minutes

Cooking time: 15 minutes

Ingredients

Cooking spray as needed

4-ounce pork loin chop, boneless and fat rimmed

1/3 cup of salsa

2 tablespoon of fresh lime juice

A ¼ cup of fresh cilantro, chopped

Directions

Take a large-sized non-stick skillet and spray it with cooking spray

Heat it up until hot over high heat

Press the chops with your palm to flatten them slightly

Add them to the skillet and cook on 1 minute for each side until they are nicely browned

Lower down the heat to medium-low

Combine the salsa and lime juice

Pour the mix over the chops

Simmer uncovered for about 8 minutes until the chops are perfectly done

If needed, sprinkle some cilantro on top

Serve!

Nutrition Values (Per Serving)

Calorie: 184

Fat: 4g

Carbohydrates: 4g

Protein: 0.5g

Smothered Pork Chops

Servings: 4

Preparation time 10 minutes

Cooking time: 30 minutes

Ingredients

4 pork chops, bone-in

2 tablespoon of olive oil

A ¼ cup of vegetable broth

½ a pound of Yukon gold potatoes, peeled and chopped

1 large onion, sliced

2 garlic cloves, minced

2 teaspoons of rubbed sage

1 teaspoon of thyme, ground

Salt and pepper as needed

Directions

Preheat your oven to 350 degrees Fahrenheit

Take a large-sized skillet and place it over medium heat

Add a tablespoon of oil and allow the oil to heat up

Add pork chops and cook them for 4-5 minutes per side until browned

Transfer chops to a baking dish

Pour broth over the chops

Add remaining oil to the pan and Sauté potatoes, onion, garlic for 3-4 minutes

Take a large bowl and add potatoes, garlic, onion, thyme, sage, pepper, and salt

Transfer this mixture to the baking dish (with pork)

Bake for 20-30 minutes

Serve and enjoy!

Nutrition Values (Per Serving)

Calorie: 261

Fat: 10g

Carbohydrates: 1.3g

Protein: 2g

Spicy Pork Chops

Servings: 4

Preparation time 4 hours 10 minutes

Cooking time: 15 minutes

Ingredients

¼ cup lime juice

4 pork rib chops

1 tablespoon coconut oil, melted

2 garlic cloves, peeled and minced

1 tablespoon chili powder

1 teaspoon ground cinnamon

2 teaspoons cumin

Salt and pepper to taste

½ teaspoon hot pepper sauce

Mango, sliced

Directions

Take a bowl and mix in lime juice, oil, garlic, cumin, cinnamon, chili powder, salt, pepper, hot pepper sauce

Whisk well

Add pork chops and toss

Keep it on the side and let it refrigerate for 4 hours

Preheat your grill to medium and transfer pork chops to a pre-heated grill

Grill for 7 minutes, flip and cook for 7 minutes more

Divide between serving platters and serve with mango slices

Enjoy!

Nutrition:

Calories: 200

Fat: 8g

Carbohydrates: 3g

Protein: 26g

Mediterranean Pork

Servings: 4

Preparation time 10 minutes

Cooking time: 35 minutes

Ingredients

4 pork chops, bone-in

Salt and pepper to taste

1 teaspoon dried rosemary

3 garlic cloves, peeled and minced

Directions

Season pork chops with salt and pepper

Place in roasting pan

Add rosemary, garlic in a pan

Preheat your oven to 425 degrees F

Bake for 10 minutes

Lower heat to 350 degrees F

Roast for 25 minutes more

Slice pork and divide on plates

Drizzle pan juice all over

Serve and enjoy!

Nutrition:

Calories: 165

Fat: 2g

Carbohydrates: 2g

Protein: 26g

Paprika Lamb Chops

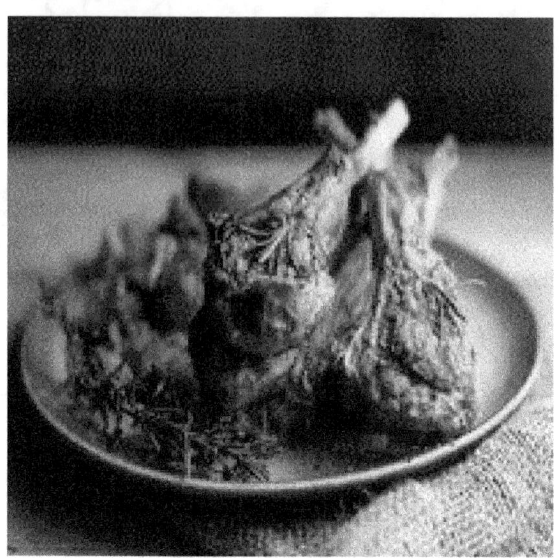

Servings: 4

Preparation time 10 minutes

Cooking time: 15 minutes

Ingredients

2 lamb racks, cut into chops

Salt and pepper to taste

3 tablespoons paprika

¾ cup cumin powder

1 teaspoon chili powder

Directions

Take a bowl and add paprika, cumin, chili, salt, pepper, and stir

Add lamb chops and rub the mixture

Heat grill over medium-temperature and add lamb chops, cook for 5 minutes

Flip and cook for 5 minutes more, flip again

Cook for 2 minutes, flip and cook for 2 minutes more

Serve and enjoy!

Nutrition:

Calories: 200

Fat: 5g

Carbohydrates: 4g

Protein: 8g

Delicious Turkey Wrap

Servings: 6

Preparation time 10 minutes

Cooking time: 10 minutes

Ingredients

1 and a ¼ pounds of ground turkey, lean

4 green onions, minced

1 tablespoon of olive oil

1 garlic clove, minced

2 teaspoons of chili paste

8-ounce water chestnut, diced

3 tablespoon of hoisin sauce

2 tablespoon of coconut aminos

1 tablespoon of rice vinegar

12 butter lettuce leaves

1/8 teaspoon of salt

Directions

Take a pan and place it over medium heat, add turkey and garlic to the pan

Heat for 6 minutes until cooked

Take a bowl and transfer turkey to the bowl

Add onions and water chestnuts

Stir in hoisin sauce, coconut aminos, vinegar, and chili paste

Toss well and transfer the mix to lettuce leaves

Serve and enjoy!

Nutrition:

Calories: 162

Fat: 4g

Net Carbohydrates: 7g

Protein: 23g

Bacon and Chicken Garlic Wrap

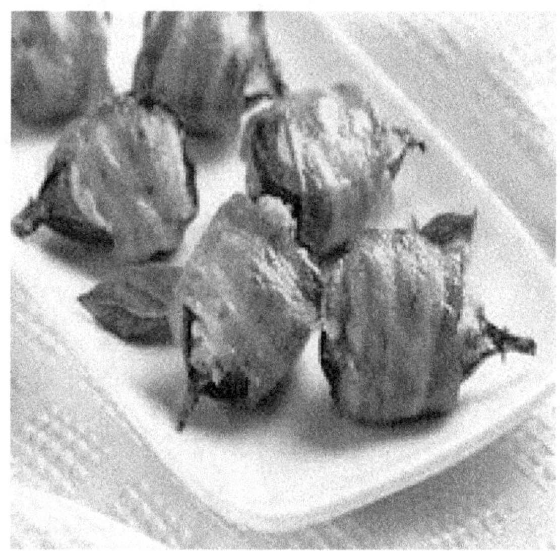

Servings: 4

Preparation time 15 minutes

Cooking time: 10 minutes

Ingredients

1 chicken fillet, cut into small cubes

8-9 thin slices bacon, cut to fit cubes

6 garlic cloves, minced

Directions

Preheat your oven to 400 degrees F

Line a baking tray with aluminum foil

Add minced garlic to a bowl and rub each chicken piece with it

Wrap bacon piece around each garlic chicken bite

Secure with toothpick

Transfer bites to the baking sheet, keeping a little bit of space between them

Bake for about 15-20 minutes until crispy

Serve and enjoy!

Nutrition:

Calories: 260

Fat: 19g

Carbohydrates: 5g

Protein: 22g

Blackened Chicken

Servings: 4

Preparation time 10 minutes

Cooking time: 10 minutes

Ingredients

½ teaspoon paprika

1/8 teaspoon salt

¼ teaspoon cayenne pepper

¼ teaspoon ground cumin

¼ teaspoon dried thyme

1/8 teaspoon ground white pepper

1/8 teaspoon onion powder

2 chicken breasts, boneless and skinless

Directions

Preheat your oven to 350 degrees Fahrenheit

Grease baking sheet

Take a cast-iron skillet and place it over high heat

Add oil and heat it up for 5 minutes until smoking hot

Take a small bowl and mix salt, paprika, cumin, white pepper, cayenne, thyme, onion powder

Oil the chicken breast on both sides and coat the breast with the spice mix

Transfer to your hot pan and cook for 1 minute per side

Transfer to your prepared baking sheet and bake for 5 minutes

Serve and enjoy!

Nutrition:

Calories: 136

Fat: 3g

Carbohydrates: 1g

Protein: 24g

Chicken Garlic Platter

Servings: 6

Preparation time 5 minutes

Cooking time: 10 minutes

Ingredients

3 large chicken breast

10-ounces spinach, frozen and drained

3-ounce mozzarella cheese, part-skim

½ a cup of roasted red peppers, cut in long strips

1 teaspoon of olive oil

2 garlic cloves, minced

Salt and pepper as needed

Directions

Preheat your oven to 400 degrees Fahrenheit

Slice 3 chicken breast lengthwise

Take a non-stick pan and grease with cooking spray

Bake for 2-3 minutes each side

Take another skillet and cook spinach and garlic in oil for 3 minutes

Place chicken on an oven pan and top with spinach, roasted peppers, and mozzarella

Bake until the cheese melted

Enjoy!

Nutrition:

Calories: 195

Fat: 7g

Net Carbohydrates: 3g

Protein: 30g

Clean Parsley and Chicken Breast

Servings: 4

Preparation time 10 minutes

Cooking time: 40 minutes

Ingredients

1 tablespoon dry parsley

1 tablespoon dry basil

4 chicken breast halves, boneless and skinless

½ teaspoon salt

½ teaspoon red pepper flakes, crushed

2 tomatoes, sliced

Directions

Preheat your oven to 350 degrees F

Take a 9x13 inch baking dish and grease it up with cooking spray

Sprinkle 1 tablespoon of parsley, 1 teaspoon of basil and spread the mixture over your baking dish

Arrange the chicken breast halves over the dish and sprinkle garlic slices on top

Take a small bowl and add 1 teaspoon parsley, 1 teaspoon of basil, salt, basil, red pepper, and mix well. Pour the mixture over the chicken breast

Top with tomato slices and cover, bake for 25 minutes

Remove the cover and bake for 15 minutes more

Serve and enjoy!

Nutrition:

Calories: 150

Fat: 4g

Carbohydrates: 4g

Protein: 25g

Balsamic Chicken

Servings: 6

Preparation time 10 minutes

Cooking time: 25 minutes

Ingredients

6 chicken breast halves, skinless and boneless

1 teaspoon garlic salt

Ground black pepper

2 tablespoons olive oil

1 onion, thinly sliced

14 and ½ ounces tomatoes, diced

½ cup balsamic vinegar

1 teaspoon dried basil

1 teaspoon dried oregano

1 teaspoon dried rosemary

½ teaspoon dried thyme

Directions

Season both sides of your chicken breasts thoroughly with pepper and garlic salt

Take a skillet and place it over medium heat

Add some oil and cook your seasoned chicken for 3-4 minutes per side until the breasts are nicely browned

Add some onion and cook for another 3-4 minutes until the onions are browned

Pour the diced up tomatoes and balsamic vinegar over your chicken and season with some rosemary, basil, thyme, and rosemary

Simmer the chicken for about 15 minutes until they are no longer pink

Take an instant-read thermometer and check if the internal temperature gives a reading of 165 degrees Fahrenheit

If yes, then you are good to go!

Nutrition:

Calories: 196

Fat: 7g

Carbohydrates: 7g

Protein: 23g

Dinner Ideas

Paprika 'n Cajun Seasoned Onion Rings

Servings: 2

Preparation time 15 minutes

Cooking time: 25 minutes

Ingredients:

1 large white onion

2 large eggs, beaten

½ teaspoon Cajun seasoning

¾ cup of almond flour

1 ½ teaspoon paprika

½ cups of coconut oil for frying

¼ cup of water

Salt and pepper to taste

Directions

Preheat a pot with oil for 8 minutes.

Peel the onion, cut off the top and slice into circles.

In a mixing bowl, combine the water and the eggs. Season with pepper and salt.

Soak the onion in the egg mixture.

In another bowl, combine the almond flour, paprika powder, Cajun seasoning, salt, and pepper.

Dredge the onion in the almond flour mixture.

Place in the pot and cook in batches until golden brown, around 8 minutes per batch.

Nutrition:

Calories: 262; Fat: 24.1g; Carbs: 3.9g; Protein: 2.8g

Creamy Kale and Mushrooms

Servings: 2

Preparation time 10 minutes

Cooking time: 15 minutes

Ingredients:

3 cloves of garlic, minced

1 onion, chopped

1 bunch kale, stems removed and leaves chopped

3 white button mushrooms, chopped

1 cup heavy cream

5 tablespoons oil

Salt and pepper to taste

Directions

Heat oil in a pot.

Sauté the garlic and onion until fragrant for 2 minutes.

Stir in mushrooms. Season with pepper and salt. Cook for 8 minutes.

Stir in kale and coconut milk. Simmer for 5 minutes.

Adjust seasoning to taste.

Nutrition:

Calories: 365; Fat: 35.5g; Carbs: 7.9g; Protein: 6.0g

Stir-Fried Buttery Mushrooms

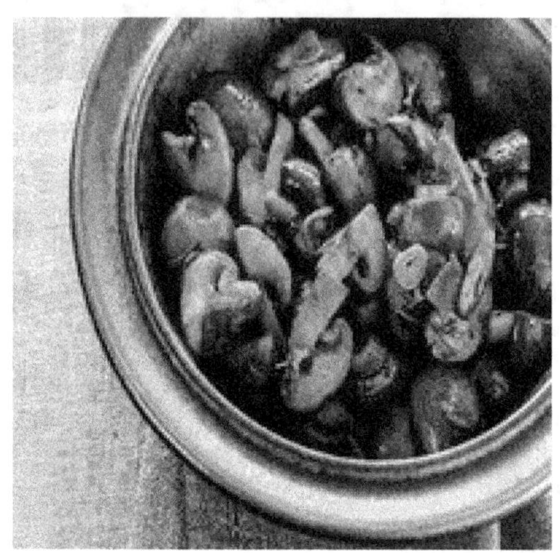

Servings: 2

Preparation time 15 minutes

Cooking time: 15 minutes

Ingredients:

4 tablespoons butter

3 cloves of garlic, minced

6 ounces' fresh brown mushrooms, sliced

7 ounces' fresh shiitake mushrooms, sliced

A dash of thyme

2 tablespoons olive oil

Salt and pepper to taste

Directions

Heat the butter and oil in a pot.

Sauté the garlic until fragrant, around 2 minutes.

Stir in the rest of the ingredients and cook until soft, around 13 minutes.

Nutrition:

Calories: 231; Fat: 17.5g; Carbs: 8.7g; Protein: 3.8g

Stir-Fried Bok Choy

Servings: 2

Preparation time minutes

Cooking time: 15 minutes

Ingredients:

4 cloves of garlic, minced

1 onion, chopped

2 heads bok choy, rinsed and chopped 2 tablespoons sesame oil

2 tablespoons sesame seeds, toasted

3 tablespoons oil

Salt and pepper to taste

Directions

Heat the oil in a pot for 2 minutes.

Sauté the garlic and onions until fragrant, around 3 minutes.

Stir in the bok choy, salt, and pepper.

Cover pan and cook for 5 minutes.

Stir and continue cooking for another 3 minutes.

Drizzle with sesame oil and sesame seeds on top before serving.

Nutrition:

Calories: 358; Fat: 28.4g; Carbs: 5.2g; Protein: 21.5g

Cauliflower Fritters

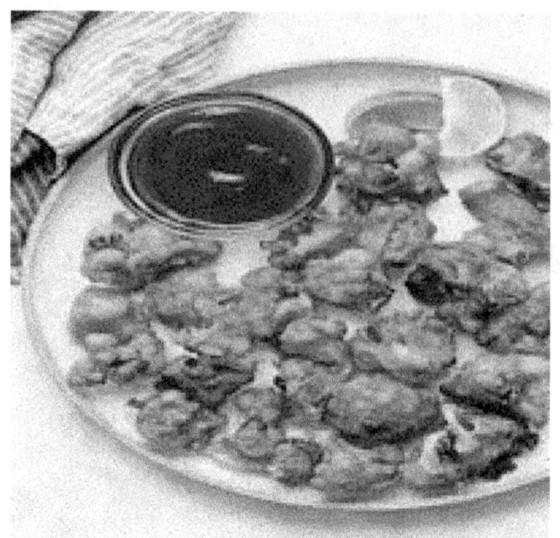

Servings: 2

Preparation time 20 minutes

Cooking time: 15 minutes

Ingredients:

1 large cauliflower head, cut into florets

2 eggs, beaten

½ teaspoon turmeric

1 large onion, peeled and chopped

½ teaspoon salt

¼ teaspoon black pepper

6 tablespoons oil

Directions

Place the cauliflower florets in a pot with water.

Bring to a boil and drain once cooked.

Place the cauliflower, eggs, onion, turmeric, salt, and pepper into the food processor.

Pulse until the mixture becomes coarse.

Transfer into a bowl. Using your hands, form six small flattened balls and place in the fridge for at least 1 hour until the mixture hardens.

Heat the oil in a skillet and fry the cauliflower patties for 3 minutes on each side.

Serve and enjoy.

Nutrition:

Calories: 157; Fat: 15.3g; Carbs: 2.28g; Protein: 3.9g

Scrambled Eggs with Mushrooms and Spinach

Servings: 2

Preparation time 3 minutes

Cooking time: 15 minutes

Ingredients:

2 large eggs

1 teaspoon butter

1/2 cup thinly sliced fresh mushrooms

1/2 cup fresh baby spinach, chopped

2 tablespoons shredded provolone cheese

1/8 teaspoon salt

1/8 teaspoon pepper

Directions

In a small bowl, whisk eggs, salt, and pepper until blended. In a small nonstick skillet, heat butter over medium-high heat. Add mushrooms; cook and stir 3-4 minutes or until tender. Add spinach; cook and stir until wilted. Reduce heat to medium.

Add egg mixture; cook and stir just until eggs are thickened, and no liquid egg remains. Stir in cheese.

Nutrition:

Calories: 162; Fat: 11g; Carbs: 2g; Protein: 14g

Endives Mix with Lemon Dressing

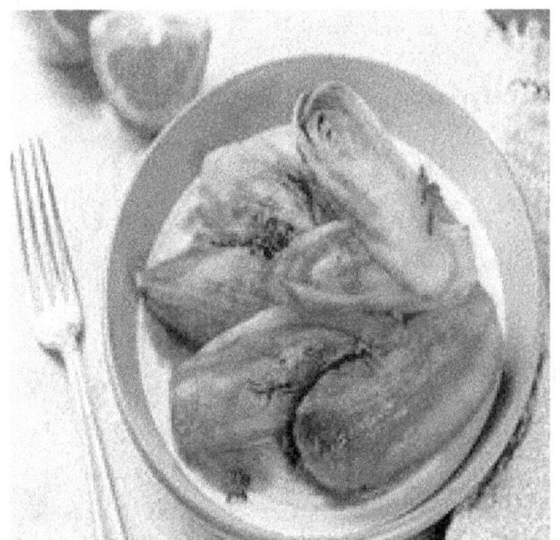

Servings: 2

Preparation time 15 minutes

Cooking time: 0 minutes

Ingredients:

1 bunch watercress (4 ounces)

2 heads endive, halved lengthwise and thinly sliced

1 cup pomegranate seeds (about 1 pomegranate)

1 shallot, thinly sliced

2 lemons, juiced and zested

1/4 teaspoon salt

1/8 teaspoon pepper

1/4 cup olive oil

Directions

In a large bowl, combine watercress, endive, pomegranate seeds, and shallot.

In a small bowl, whisk the lemon juice, zest, salt, pepper, and olive oil. Drizzle over salad; toss to coat.

Nutrition:

Calories: 151; Fat:13g; Carbs: 6g; Protein: 2g

Grilled Parmesan Eggplant

Servings: 2

Preparation time 5 minutes

Cooking time: 15 minutes

Ingredients:

1 medium-sized eggplant

1 log (1 pound) fresh mozzarella cheese, cut into sixteen slices

1 small tomato, cut into eight slices

1/2 cup shredded Parmesan cheese

Chopped fresh basil or parsley

1/2 teaspoon salt

1 tablespoon olive oil

1/2 teaspoon pepper

Directions

Trim ends of the eggplant; cut eggplant crosswise into eight slices. Sprinkle with salt; let stand 5 minutes.

Blot eggplant dry with paper towels; brush both sides with oil and sprinkle with pepper. Grill, covered, over medium heat 4-6 minutes on each side or until tender. Remove from grill.

Top eggplant with mozzarella cheese, tomato, and Parmesan cheese. Grill, covered, 1-2 minutes longer or until cheese begins to melt. Top with basil.

Nutrition:

Calories: 449; Fat: 31g; Carbs: 10g; Protein: 26g

Creamy Artichoke and Spinach

Servings: 2

Preparation time 5 minutes

Cooking time: 0 minutes

Ingredients:

5 tablespoons olive oil

1 can (8 ounces) water-packed artichoke hearts quartered

1 package (3 ounces) frozen spinach

1 cup shredded part-skim mozzarella cheese, divided

1/4 cup grated Parmesan cheese

1/2 teaspoon salt

1/4 teaspoon pepper

Directions

Heat oil in a pan over medium flame. Add artichoke hearts and season with salt and pepper to taste. Cook for 5 minutes. Stir in the spinach until wilted.

Place in a bowl and stir in mozzarella cheese, Parmesan cheese, salt, and pepper. Toss to combine.

Transfer to a greased 2-qt. Broiler-safe baking dish; sprinkle with remaining mozzarella cheese. Broil 4-6 in. from heat 2-3 minutes or until cheese is melted.

Nutrition:

Calories: 283; Fat: 23.9g; Carbs: 7.3g; Protein: 11.5g

Egg and Tomato Salad

Servings: 2

Preparation time 20 minutes

Cooking time: 1 minute

Ingredients:

4 hard-boiled eggs, peeled and sliced

2 red tomatoes, chopped

1 small red onion, chopped

2 tablespoons lemon juice, freshly squeezed

Salt and pepper to taste

4 tablespoons olive oil

Directions

Place all ingredients in a mixing bowl.

Toss to coat all ingredients.

Garnish with parsley if desired.

Serve over toasted whole wheat bread.

Nutrition:

Calories: 189; Fat: 15.9g; Carbs: 9.1g; Protein: 14.7g

Curried Tofu

Servings: 2

Preparation time 5 minutes

Cooking time: 15 minutes

Ingredients:

2 cloves of garlic, minced

1 onion, cubed

12-ounce firm tofu, drained and cubed

1 teaspoon curry powder

1 tablespoon soy sauce

¼ teaspoon pepper

5 tablespoons olive oil

Directions

Heat the oil in a skillet over medium flame.

Sauté the garlic and onion until fragrant.

Stir in the tofu and stir for 3 minutes.

Add the rest of the ingredients and adjust the water.

Close the lid and allow simmering for 10 minutes.

Serve and enjoy.

Nutrition:

Calories: 148; Fat: 14.1g; Carbs: 4.4g; Protein: 6.2g

Desserts and Snacks Ideas

Cheese Mug

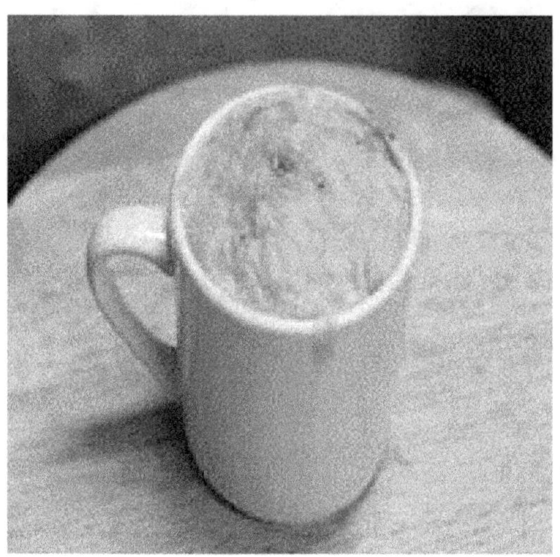

Serving: 1

Preparation time 4 minutes

Cooking time: 1-2 minutes

Ingredients

2 ounces roast beef slices

1 and ½ tablespoons green chilies, diced

1 and ½ ounces pepper jack cheese, shredded

1 tablespoon sour cream

Directions

Layer roast beef on the bottom of your mug, making sure to break it down into small pieces

Add half a tablespoon of sour cream, add half tablespoon green Chile and half an ounce of pepper jack cheese

Keep layering until all ingredients are used

Microwave for 2 minutes

Server warm and enjoy!

Nutrition:

Calories: 268

Fat: 16g

Carbohydrates: 4g

Protein: 22g

Lemon Broccoli

Servings: 4

Preparation time 10 minutes

Cooking time: 15 minutes

Ingredients

2 heads broccoli, separated into florets

2 teaspoons extra virgin olive oil

1 teaspoon salt

½ teaspoon pepper

1 garlic clove, minced

½ teaspoon lemon juice

Directions

Preheat your oven to a temperature of 400 degrees F

Take a large-sized bowl and add broccoli florets with some extra virgin olive oil, pepper, sea salt and garlic

Spread the broccoli out in a single even layer on a fine baking sheet

Bake in your pre-heated oven for about 15-20 minutes until the florets are soft enough so that they can be pierced with a fork

Squeeze lemon juice over them generously before serving

Enjoy!

Nutrition:

Calories: 49

Fat: 2g

Carbohydrates: 4g

Protein: 3g

Coconut Candy

Serving: 1

Preparation time 10 minutes

Cooking Time: 0 minutes

Ingredients:

2-tbsp coconut butter (or notably known as Coconut Manna)

Directions:

Melt the coconut butter at room temperature until it resembles a creamy butter consistency.

Spoon out the melted butter into candy molds. Refrigerate for 10 minutes to harden before serving.

Nutrition:

Calories: 204

Fat: 17.2g Protein: 10.2g Total Carbohydrates: 3g Dietary Fiber: 0.8g Net Carbohydrates: 2.2g

Mozzarella Mound Munchies

Servings: 3

Preparation time 5 minutes

Cooking Time: 6 minutes

Ingredients:

⅓-cup panko bread, herb-flavored

2-pcs egg whites

6-tbsp mozzarella cheese, molded into 2-tbsp balls

¼-cup marinara sauce

Directions:

Preheat your oven to 425°F.

Toast the panko breadcrumbs for 2 minutes, frequently stirring, in a medium skillet placed over medium heat.

Transfer the breadcrumbs in a bowl. Add the egg whites into a separate bowl.

Dip a cheeseball into the egg and roll in the panko. Place the breaded cheese on a greased baking sheet, and bake for 3 minutes. Repeat the process for the remaining cheese.

Heat the marinara sauce in your microwave oven for half a minute. Serve the breaded cheeseball with the sauce

Nutrition:

Calories: 157

Fat: 13.2g

Protein: 5.9g

Total Carbohydrates: 4.8g

Dietary Fiber: 1.1g

Net Carbohydrates: 3.7g

Philadelphia Potato Praline

Servings: 2

Preparation time 30 minutes

Cooking Time: 0 minutes

Ingredients:

⅓-cup Philadelphia cream cheese

1½-cup coconut, unsweetened and shredded

1-tbsp butter

¼-tsp ground cinnamon

Sweetener of choice

Directions:

Mix all the ingredients apart from ground cinnamon in a bowl. Refrigerate the mixture and allow the setting until it hardens.

Divide the mixture into 8 and roll each portion into potato shapes. Place them on a sheet of parchment paper.

Sprinkle all over with the cinnamon and store in the fridge for a week before serving.

Nutrition:

Calories: 180

Fat: 15.3g

Protein: 8.9g

Total Carbohydrates: 3.2g

Dietary Fiber: 1.5g

Net Carbohydrates: 1.7g

Tasty Turkey Cheese Cylinders

Serving: 1

Preparation time 5 minutes

Cooking Time: 0 minutes

Ingredients:

1-oz. turkey, roasted and sliced

1-oz. cheese

Directions:

Slice the cheese into a long strip, enough to fit the turkey slice.

Wrap the turkey slice around the cheese.

Nutrition:

Calories: 162

Fat: 10.9g

Protein: 15.6g

Total Carbohydrates: 3.8g

Dietary Fiber: 0g

Net Carbohydrates: 3.8g

Fried Flaxseed Tortilla Treat

Servings: 3

Preparation time 5 minutes

Cooking Time: 10 minutes

Ingredients:

6-shells flaxseed tortillas, sliced into chip-sized cuts

3-tbsp olive oil

A dash of salt and pepper

Directions:

Fry the flaxseed chips with olive oil in a large pan placed over medium-high heat. Cook for 10 minutes until the chips become crispy, stirring frequently. Strain the chips and place them on a paper towel to drain excess oil.

Season with salt and pepper.

Nutrition:

Calories: 36

Fat: 2.8g

Protein: 0.8g

Total Carbohydrates: 2.7g

Dietary Fiber: 0.7g

Net Carbohydrates: 2g

Kingly Kale Crispy Chips

Serving: 1

Prep time:4 minutes

Cooking Time: 12 minutes

Ingredients

1-bunch large kale, rinsed, drained, and stemless

2-tbsp olive oil

1-tbsp salt

Directions:

Preheat your oven to 350°F.

Place the kale in a plastic bag. Pour the oil, and mix well by shaking the bag until coating thoroughly each leaf.

Spread the kale onto a baking sheet. Press the leaves flat to obtain an evenly crisped cook for each leaf.

Bake for 12 minutes until the edges turn brown while the rest of the kales remain dark green.

Sprinkle the salt over the baked kale and serve.

Nutrition:

Calories: 110

Fat: 28g

Protein:8g

Total Carbohydrates: 18g

Dietary Fiber: 8g

Net Carbohydrates: 3g

Ambrosial Avocado Puree Pudding

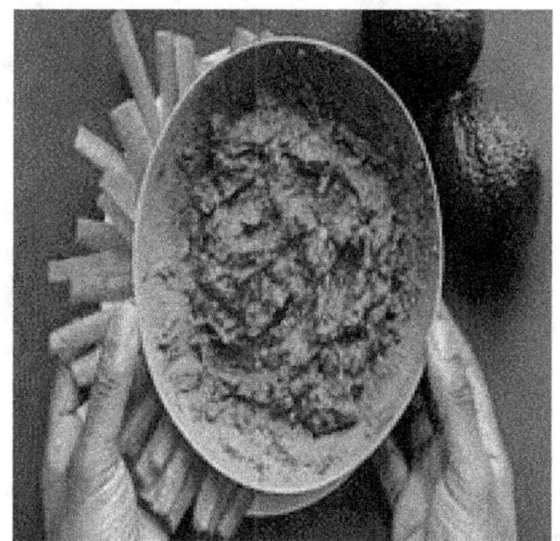

Servings: 3

Preparation time 5 minutes

Cooking Time: 0 minutes

Ingredients

2-ripe Hass avocados, peeled, pitted and cut into chunks

2-tsp organic vanilla extract

80-drops of liquid sweetener

1-can (113.5-oz.) organic coconut milk

1-tbsp lime juice from organic lime

Directions

Combine all the ingredients in a blender. Blend to a smooth and velvety consistency. Pour the blend equally between three glasses. Chill before serving.

Nutrition:

Calories: 240

Fat: 23.8g

Protein: 2.8g

Total Carbohydrates: 12.8g

Dietary Fiber: 9g

Net Carbohydrates: 3.8g

Power-Packed Butter Balls

Servings: 5

Preparation time 80 minutes

Cooking Time: 0 minutes

Ingredients:

2-tbsp cocoa powder + 1-tbsp for dusting

2-tbsp plain oatmeal, gluten-free

⅔-cup peanut butter or chia butter

1-tbsp organic chia seeds

3-tbsp protein powder

Directions:

Mix the cocoa powder, oatmeal, peanut butter chia seeds, and protein powder.

By using your hand, form balls from the mixture. Dust each ball with cocoa powder.

Place the balls in the fridge for 1 hour before serving.

Nutrition:

Calories: 128

Fat: 10.1g

Protein: 4.9g

Total Carbohydrates: 7.2g

Dietary Fiber: 2.9g

Net Carbohydrates: 4.3g

Choco Coco Cups

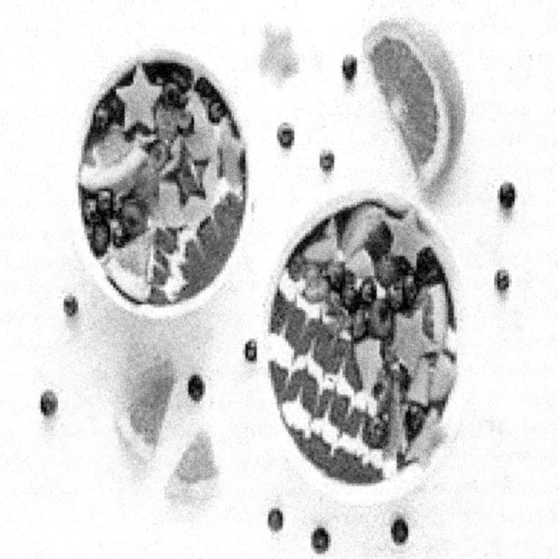

Servings: 10

Preparation time 50 minutes

Cooking Time: 0 minutes

Ingredients:

For the Coconut Base:

½-cup coconut butter

½-cup coconut oil

½-cup unsweetened coconut, shredded

3-tbsp powdered sweetener

For the Chocolate Topping:

3-oz. sugar-free dark chocolate

Directions:

Line a muffin pan with 20 mini parchment cups.

Heat the coconut butter with the coconut oil in a saucepan placed over low heat. Stir until the butter melts. Stir in the sweetener and coconut and sweetener until fully combined.

Divide the mixture equally between the prepared muffin cups. Freeze for 30 minutes until firm.

Melt the dark chocolate and spoon over the cold filling. Let it sit for 15 minutes before serving.

Nutrition:

Calories: 240

Fat: 25.3g

Protein: 2.1g

Total Carbohydrates: 5g

Dietary Fiber: 4g

Net Carbohydrates: 1g

Corndog Clumps

Servings: 10

Preparation time 5 minutes

Cooking Time: 15 minutes

Ingredients:

¼-tsp. baking powder

¼-tsp. salt

½-cup almond flour

½-cup flaxseed meal

1-tbsp psyllium husk powder

3-packets sweetener

1-pc large egg

⅓-cup sour cream

¼-cup melted butter

¼-cup coconut milk

10-pcs (2-oz.) smoked sausage, sliced in half

Directions:

Preheat your oven to 375°F. Grease a 20-cup muffin pan.

Combine the first six ingredients in a bowl. Add the egg, sour cream, and butter and mix well. Pour in the coconut milk and mix again. Pour the batter in the pan.

Insert a sliced sausage into the center of each muffin. Place the pan in the oven.

Bake for 12 minutes; thereafter, broil for 3 minutes, set on high heat.

Nutrition:

Calories: 148

Fat: 13.2g

Protein: 3.9g

Total Carbohydrates: 4g

Dietary Fiber: 1.6g

Net Carbohydrates: 3.4g

Stuffed Mushrooms

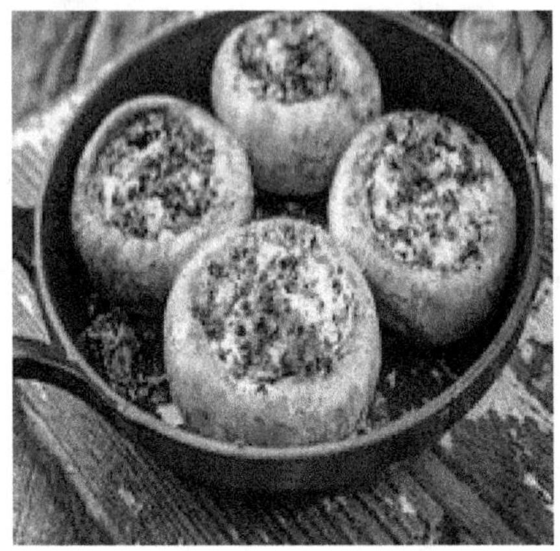

Servings: 4

Preparation time 10 minutes

Cooking time: 15 minutes

Ingredients

4 Portobello mushrooms

1 cup crumbled blue cheese

2 teaspoons extra virgin olive oil

Salt, to taste

Fresh thyme

Directions

Preheat your oven to 350 degrees Fahrenheit

Put out the stems from the mushrooms

Chop them into small pieces

Take a bowl and mix stem pieces with thyme, salt, and blue cheese and mix well

Fill up mushroom with the prepared cheese

Top them with some oil

Take a baking sheet and place the mushrooms

Bake for 15 minutes to 20 minutes

Serve warm and enjoy!

Nutrition:

Calories: 124

Fat: 22.4g

Carbohydrates: 5.4g

Protein: 1.2g

Garlic Bread Stick

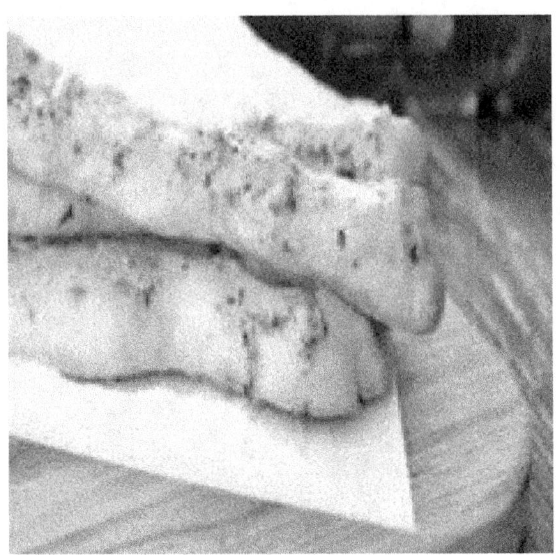

Servings: 8 breadsticks

Preparation time 15 minutes

Cooking time: 15 minutes

Ingredients

¼ cup butter softened

1 teaspoon garlic powder

2 cups almond flour

½ tablespoon baking powder

1 tablespoon Psyllium husk powder

¼ teaspoon salt

3 tablespoons butter, melted

1 egg

¼ cup boiling water

Directions

Preheat your oven to 400 degrees F

Line baking sheet with parchment paper and keep it on the side

Beat butter with garlic powder and keep it on the side

Add almond flour, baking powder, husk, salt in a bowl and mix in butter and egg, mix well

Pour boiling water in the mix and stir until you have a nice dough

Divide the dough into 8 balls and roll into breadsticks

Place on a baking sheet and bake for 15 minutes

Brush each stick with garlic butter and bake for 5 minutes more

Serve and enjoy!

Nutrition:

Calories: 259

Fat: 24g

Carbohydrates: 5g

Protein: 7g

Camembert Mushrooms

Servings: 4

Preparation time 5 minutes

Cooking time: 13 minutes

Ingredients

2 tablespoons butter

4 ounces Camembert cheese, diced

2 teaspoons garlic, minced

1 pound button mushrooms, halved

Black pepper to taste

Directions

Place a skillet over medium-high heat

Add butter and let it melt

Once the butter has melted, add garlic and Sauté until translucent, should take 3 minutes

Add mushrooms and cook for 10 minutes

Season with pepper and serve

Enjoy!

Nutrition:

Calories: 161

Fat: 13g

Carbohydrates: 3g

Protein: 9g

Eggplant Fries

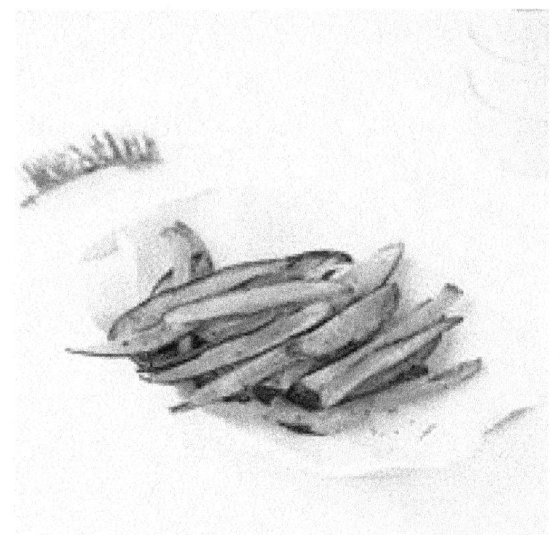

Servings: 8

Preparation time 10 minutes

Cooking time: 15 minutes

Ingredients

2 eggs

2 cups almond flour

2 tablespoons coconut oil, spray

2 eggplants, peeled and cut thinly

Salt and pepper

Directions

Preheat your oven to 400 degrees Fahrenheit

Take a bowl and mix with salt and black pepper in it

Take another bowl and beat eggs until frothy

Dip the eggplant pieces into eggs

Then coat them with flour mixture

Add another layer of flour and egg

Then, take a baking sheet and grease with coconut oil on top

Bake for about 15 minutes

Serve and enjoy!

Nutrition:

Calories: 212

Fat: 15.8g

Carbohydrates: 12.1g

Protein: 8.6g

Parmesan Crisps

Servings: 8

Preparation time 5 minutes

Cooking time: 25 minutes

Ingredients

1 teaspoon butter

8 ounces' parmesan cheese, full fat and shredded

Directions

Preheat your oven to 400 degrees F

Put parchment paper on a baking sheet and grease with butter

Spoon parmesan into 8 mounds, spreading them apart evenly

Flatten them

Bake for 5 minutes until browned

Let them cool

Serve and enjoy!

Nutrition:

Calories: 133

Fat: 11g

Carbohydrates: 1g

Protein: 11g

Roasted Broccoli

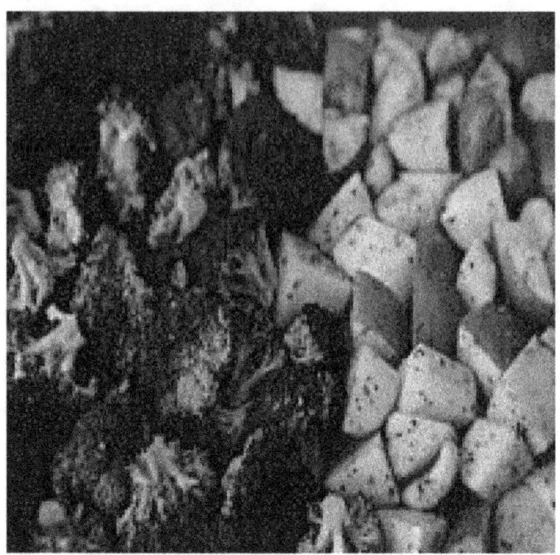

Servings: 4

Preparation time 5 minutes

Cooking time: 20 minutes

Ingredients

4 cups broccoli florets

1 tablespoon olive oil

Salt and pepper to taste

Directions

Preheat your oven to 400 degrees F

Add broccoli in a zip bag alongside oil and shake until coated

Add seasoning and shake again

Spread broccoli out on the baking sheet, bake for 20 minutes

Let it cool and serve

Enjoy!

Nutrition:

Calories: 62

Fat: 4g

Carbohydrates: 4g

Protein: 4g

Lemon Mousse

Preparation time:10 minutes

Servings: 2

Ingredients:

14 oz coconut milk

12 drops liquid stevia

1/2 tsp lemon extract

1/4 tsp turmeric

Directions:

Place coconut milk can in the refrigerator overnight. Scoop out thick cream into a mixing bowl.

Add remaining ingredients to the bowl and whip using a hand mixer until smooth.

Transfer mousse mixture to a zip lock bag and pipe into small serving glasses. Place in refrigerator.

Serve chilled and enjoy.

Nutrition:

Calories 444;

Fat 45.7 g;

Carbohydrates 10 g;

Sugar 6 g;

Protein 4.4 g;

Cholesterol 0 mg;

Avocado Pudding

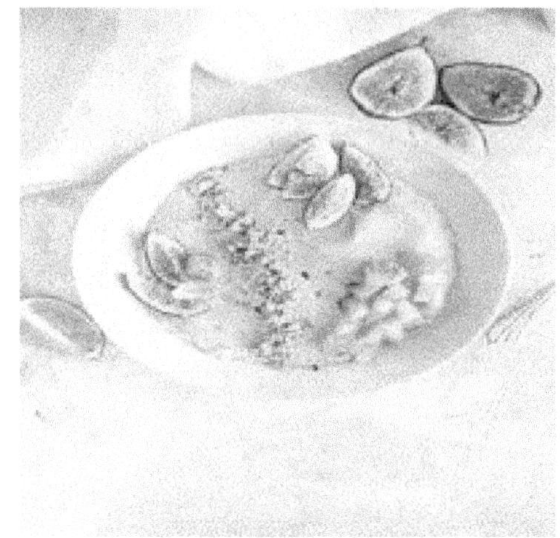

Servings: 8

Preparation time:10 minutes

Ingredients:

2 ripe avocados, peeled, pitted and cut into pieces

1 tbsp fresh lime juice

14 oz can coconut milk

80 drops of liquid stevia

2 tsp vanilla extract

Directions:

Add all ingredients into the blender and blend until smooth.
Serve and enjoy.

Nutrition:

Calories 317;

Fat 30.1 g;

Carbohydrates 9.3 g;

Sugar 0.4 g;

Protein 3.4 g;

Cholesterol 0 mg;

Almond Butter Brownies

Preparation time:30 minutes

Servings: 4

Ingredients:

1 scoop protein powder

2 tbsp cocoa powder

1/2 cup almond butter, melted

1 cup bananas, overripe

Directions:

Preheat the oven to 350 F/ 176 C.

Spray brownie tray with cooking spray.

Add all ingredients into the blender and blend until smooth.

Pour batter into the prepared dish and bake in preheated oven for 20 minutes.

Serve and enjoy.

Nutrition:

Calories 82;

Fat 2.1 g;

Carbohydrates 11.4 g;

Protein 6.9 g;

Sugars 5 g;

Cholesterol 16 mg;

Chocolate Fudge

Preparation time:10 minutes

Servings: 12

Ingredients:

4 oz unsweetened dark chocolate

3/4 cup coconut butter

15 drops liquid stevia

1 tsp vanilla extract

Directions:

Melt coconut butter and dark chocolate.

Add ingredients to the large bowl and combine well.

Pour mixture into a silicone loaf pan and place it in the refrigerator until set.

Cut into pieces and serve.

Nutrition:

Calories 157;

Fat 14.1 g;

Carbohydrates 6.1 g;

Sugar 1 g;

Protein 2.3 g;

Cholesterol 0 mg;

Coconut Peanut Butter Fudge

Preparation time:1 hour 15 minutes

Servings: 20

Ingredients:

12 oz smooth peanut butter

3 tbsp coconut oil

4 tbsp coconut cream

15 drops liquid stevia

Pinch of salt

Directions:

Line baking tray with parchment paper.

Melt coconut oil in a saucepan over low heat.

Add peanut butter, coconut cream, stevia, and salt in a saucepan. Stir well.

Pour fudge mixture into the prepared baking tray and place it in the refrigerator for 1 hour.

Cut into pieces and serve.

Nutrition:

Calories 125;

Fat 11.3 g;

Carbohydrates 3.5 g;

Sugar 1.7 g;

Protein 4.3 g;

Cholesterol 0 mg;

Raspberry Chia Pudding

Preparation time:3 hours 10 minutes

Servings: 2

Ingredients:

4 tbsp chia seeds

1 cup of coconut milk

1/2 cup raspberries

Directions:

Add raspberry and coconut milk in a blender and blend until smooth.

Pour mixture into the Mason jar.

Add chia seeds in a jar and stir well.

Close the jar tightly with lid and shake well.

Place in the refrigerator for 3 hours.

Serve chilled and enjoy.

Nutrition:

Calories 361;

Fat 33.4 g;

Carbohydrates 13.3 g;

Sugar 5.4 g;

Protein 6.2 g;

Cholesterol 0 mg;

Quick Chocó Brownie

Preparation time:10 minutes

Serving: 1

Ingredients:

1/4 cup almond milk

1 tbsp cocoa powder

1 scoop chocolate protein powder

1/2 tsp baking powder

Directions:

In a microwave-safe mug, blend together baking powder, protein powder, and cocoa.

Add almond milk in a mug and stir well.

Place mug in microwave and microwave for 30 seconds.

Serve and enjoy.

Nutrition:

Calories 207;

Fat 15.8 g;

Carbohydrates 9.5 g;

Sugar 3.1 g;

Protein 12.4 g;

Cholesterol 20 mg;

Chocó Chia Pudding

Preparation time:10 minutes

Servings: 6

Ingredients:

2 1/2 cups coconut milk

2 scoops stevia extract powder

6 tbsp cocoa powder

1/2 cup of chia seeds

1/2 tsp vanilla extract

1/8 cup of xylitol

1/8 tsp salt

Directions:

Add all ingredients into the blender and blend until smooth.

Pour mixture into the glass container and place it in the refrigerator.

Serve chilled and enjoy.

Nutrition:

Calories 259;

Fat 25.4 g;

Carbohydrates 10.2 g;

Sugar 3.5 g;

Protein 3.8 g;

Cholesterol 0 mg;

Smooth Chocolate Mousse

Preparation time:10 minutes

Servings: 2

Ingredients:

1/2 tsp cinnamon

3 tbsp unsweetened cocoa powder

1 cup creamed coconut milk

10 drops liquid stevia

Directions:

Place coconut milk can in the refrigerator overnight; it should get thick and the solids separate from water.

Transfer thick part into the large mixing bowl without water.

Add remaining ingredients to the bowl and whip with an electric mixer until smooth.

Serve and enjoy.

Nutrition: Calories 296; Fat 29.7 g; Carbohydrates

11.5 g; Sugar 4.2 g; Protein 4.4 g; Cholesterol 0 mg;

Chapter 7: Final Tips and Tricks

Set Your Goals

Before you decide to start a diet, it is time to analyze why you want to start a diet. What are the reasons why you wish to diet? What are your goals? You might want to lose weight, improve your fitness levels, or even lead a healthier life. Reasons tend to vary from one individual to another. If you don't set any goals for yourself, you will quickly lose motivation after a couple of weeks of dieting. However, while setting goals. There are a couple of simple things you must keep in mind. Ensure that the goals you set are specific, measurable, attainable, relevant, and time-bound. Even if one of these ingredients is missing, then the chances of attaining such a goal will reduce.

If you set any unrealistic goals for yourself, you are setting yourself up for failure. For instance, a goal like, "I want to lose 40 pounds within four weeks," is quite unrealistic. By setting such lofty goals, you are setting yourself up for failure. When you cannot attain such an impossible goal, you will be demotivated, and you will quickly lose interest in dieting altogether. Any goal that you set needs to have a time limit. If you don't set a time limit for yourself, procrastination can creep in, and the likelihood of sticking to the diet will also reduce. Therefore, an ideal goal would be, "I want to lose two to three pounds every month."

Pick a date

You must always pick a date to start this diet. Don't be in a hurry and think that you can get started with this diet right away. There are a couple of things you need to do before you can begin to diet. For instance, you will need to stock up on all the ingredients you require to cook keto-friendly meals. Apart from this, you will also need to prepare yourself mentally to get started with the new diet. All this takes planning and preparation. You cannot skip these two necessary steps if you want to stick to the diet in the long run. When you opt for a specific date, ensure that you start dieting, from that day itself. Don't procrastinate, and don't tell yourself that you can start dieting from tomorrow. That "tomorrow" might never have come around. Maybe you can mark the date on your calendar to remind yourself that you are supposed to start with your diet.

Meal Plan

To ensure that you stick to the diet, you will need a meal plan. The good news is you don't have to create a meal plan for yourself. There is a detailed meal plan in this book. You can use it to get started with your new diet. Ensure that you include plenty of variety. Whenever you plan, the meals out for a week. If the food you eat starts getting repetitive, you will quickly lose interest to stick to your diet. Also, when you have a meal plan in place, it becomes easier to shop for groceries. If you know that you have a healthy meal waiting for you at home, the temptation of eating out will also reduce.

Make Calories Count

A common reason why a lot of people lose interest in dieting is because of hunger pangs. Ensure that you make every calorie count. Don't binge on unhealthy foods and instead, opt for nutrient-dense options. When your tummy is full, the urge to snack on junk food will reduce. If your daily calorie intake is 1800 calories, then ensure that you manage to eat at least two well-balanced, hearty meals. You can undoubtedly blow this calorie count by binging on a pint of ice cream, but it will do you no good.

Grocery Shopping

It is time to clean your pantry! Raid your kitchen and discard any unhealthy foods you find. Get rid of all cookies, cakes, chocolates, sodas, and other foods you must not eat while on the keto diet. Out of sight and out of mind is the best policy when it comes to dieting. If temptations surround you, the urge to give in will increase. Instead, stock up your pantry will keto-friendly ingredients. Once you have all the ingredients you need, it becomes easier to cook as well. Always prepare a grocery list before you go shopping and stick to this list.

Visualization

Whenever you are running low on motivation, remind yourself of the reasons why you started dieting. Think about the goals you want to attain. Start visualizing your goals. Think about how wonderful and happy you will feel when you attain your goals.

While doing this, also think about how disappointed you would be if you didn't attain those same goals. While visualizing your goals, try to make the visualization as detailed as you possibly can. If you want, you can create a visualization board for yourself. Take a sheet of paper, make a note of your goal on it, and place it somewhere visible. Glance at it daily. It will act as a subconscious reminder for your mind. Fill this board up with positive affirmations, quotes, or even images that motivate you to stick to the diet.

A Dieting Buddy

The best way to ensure that you stay on track and stick to your diet is to find a dieting partner for yourself. Maybe you can start this diet with your partner, a friend, a loved one, family member, or anyone else. If you want, there are plenty of online forums; you can join and interact with others who are going through the same situation that you are in. When you do this, you will realize that you aren't alone. This, by itself, will give you plenty of motivation to keep going.

By following the simple tips given in this section, you can ensure that your motivation levels stay high as you get started with this diet.

Ride out the Hunger Waves

Pangs of hunger do not endure for a long time, but they can be harrowing. But the moment they emerge, they can be intolerable so you can resort to huger waves. Opposite of the popular opinion that when hunger comes up, it eats up you inside more and more till you sense death, but it subsides depending on the way you can make it through. When someone is hungry, what happens to their body is hydration. a particular body may exhibit dehydration by having symptoms of hunger when what needs to be done is just take a cup of water.

Start Gradually

When embarking on a new lifestyle or grappling with intermittent fasting, the food advice is to do it gradually. Everybody needs time to adapt and transition itself without haste. For instance, if you are fasting through the normal dinner time until six in the morning, make sure you see yourself through without any food around, even the ensuing day, even stretching up to lunchtime. Some folks have the inclination to get into anything new without any forethought, and they push themselves through the hard spans of times and cravings. But the best of all gradual conveniences process is the best way to travel no matter how rocky it is. In conclusion, we can draw a lot from intermittent fasting; also, we should not have unfounded expectations from weight loss, good body posture no matter how strict the fasting path might be.

Meanwhile, there will be jiffies of weight loss, as the body's systems funnel itself to the trials. But everything will most likely change eventually after the fasting period. This can be visible during the initial weeks of transition as the body will be trying cling on to everything that to the time it figures itself out. But the time it figures the process, later on, everything will come to join the dotted path to follow through. Every diet is meant to have weight gains or loss paradigm. This could be part of weight gain or loss, and it cannot be controlled. But there are consistent and feasible measures that will prove adaptable and workable, but the futile thing is to try to change things up whimsically because this can spiral into a more problematic conundrum of events. Whereas if you pursue a positive course and exert oneself to the good work, the fine results will be eminent and visible before you come to realize.

Always bear in mind any strenuous physical activity requires precautions in the same case our intermittent fasting needs lot care because our very souls are involved and depend on it. The health benefits cannot be underestimated because it can prevent diseases and enhance spiritual wellbeing. Even those who are overweight can help to cut down the body mass as well. There are those with eating disorders, so they should not strenuously exert themselves on it. So in hindsight, timing your meals can improve your wellbeing, control weight, and, most of all, make you physically active. So the resolve to achieve better results is good regardless of distractions one has to encounter along the way, but the payback will be worth pursuing.

Adjust Your Diet Plan as You Go

I shared an excellent diet plan with you in this book, and it is perfectly normal and okay to follow the plan for the full two weeks that I have designed it for. Even after that, you may continue with the program in order to experience more benefits, such as reduced body weight and to gain an improvement in your overall health.

Now, at the same time, I do want to note that following one single plan over an extended period will often not offer you the best results that you could achieve through intermittent fasting.

The thing is every person is different – you are unique. For this reason, a specific meal plan that works for you will likely not be ideal for every single person.

This means that the diet program that I introduced you in this book might be able to work, but you may need to make some modifications as you go along to achieve the specific goals that you have in mind with the program that you are implementing.

Sure, you are not a dietician with years of experience in the industry, which does make it somewhat harder for you to develop an appropriate diet plan that will suit you and help you achieve the goals you are striving toward. This, however, does not necessarily mean that it will be impossible for you to make simple adjustments in order to reach those weight loss goals.

Don't Overlook The Importance Of Exercise In a Weight-Loss Strategy

You should have read the topic where I explained how intermittent fasting is used for weight loss already by now, so you should understand that without expending calories each day, you won't be able to lose that excess fat that has accumulated inside your body.

Expending calories mean being physically active. Unfortunately, quite a large percentage of the worldwide population are living sedentary lifestyles. With a sedentary lifestyle, you are really "paving the way" for weight gain. If you are not physically active, you won't be able to burn an adequate number of calories each day for weight loss to be possible in the first place.

The more you exercise, the more calories you will burn, of course. At the same time, you should be sure not to overdo things in terms of physical activity. There is no use in causing yourself injury due to overtraining – this will only lead to temporary disability and will make training harder for the next few days (sometimes weeks or months if you suffer a more serious injury).

It is best to create a balanced exercise plan for yourself and then test it out. Listen to your body and understand when you are pushing yourself, as well as when you have some extra capacity available to up your game at the gym.

You will have to take your daily calorie consumption into account here – we did discuss how you can calculate your ideal daily calorie requirement in a previous section. This data will definitely come in handy here. Calculate an appropriate exercise plan that will ensure your daily caloric expenditure reached through physical exercise will reach past your daily caloric intake.

Deal with Hunger Pangs Like a Boss

Let's tackle a topic that you will likely face yourself. Hunger pangs are something that we all experience when we first start with an intermittent fasting plan. You suddenly have to get your body adjusted to an entirely new way of eating. No longer do you get up in the morning and cook up some eggs and bacon. You have to get up and drink water, or perhaps have a cup of coffee, but you'll have to wait until the afternoon before you get to have your first meal.

So, the question now is, should you give in to the temptations that you will be experiencing, especially during those first few days, or should you implement an appropriate strategy to help you better cope with these hunger pangs and the cravings that you are going to experience.

There are different strategies that you can use to cope with your cravings. One would be to drink a glass of water if you feel hungry, and you can feel those cravings building up. This is an effective strategy for lots of people, but not for everyone, of course. If you find that plain water or even filtered water does not work well for you, then I suggest you try some fizzy water (carbonated water). Be sure not to opt for carbonated water with added sweetening agents, as these are loaded with some carbs. Rather just opt for plain sparkling water. The carbonation in the water can help to make you feel full for a while to ensure you can get through to your eating window without giving in to your temptations.

It is important that you are patient and practice self-control when cravings start building up. Giving in to these cravings should not be considered okay now-and-then, as this will break the fasting window, and it will yield less effective results compared to ensuring you last until you are inside of your eating window.

Physical Activity

Like meal planning, measuring foods, reading food labels, and portion control, exercise is NOT required, but beneficial to your overall results while doing intermittent fasting. The American Heart Association recommends some form of physical activity for at least 30 minutes daily.

Create a workout schedule. Make a leg day, an arms day, cardio day, total body weight day, and more. A schedule starts to make you more consistent and accountable. On days when you feel unmotivated to do one, you have the other. If you are already exercising, intermittent fasting can only improve your results. The combination of intermittent fasting and exercise maximizes weight loss and/or weight maintenance.

Mindset

The biggest barrier, if any, will be your mindset. The barrier will be the already set attitudes and assumptions you have in your head, specifically as it relates to the relationship you have with food and eating food. Think mind over matter, and you matter the most to yourself, so take better care of yourself. To sustain following an intermittent lifestyle, you will need to erase or ignore all prior assumptions or attitudes related to diets/lifestyle changes, losing weight, current food habits, current eating schedules, changes in general, and more. Once started, try to make optimal choices for yourself and be disciplined in being consistent in carrying out your plans. To be successful, you will need to think and act differently for optimal results.

Conclusion

Whether you are only overweight or have already reached the point where you are considered obese, excess weight in the body can lead to several adverse health effects that can eventually cause life-threatening conditions to develop. When excess fat accumulates, weight loss becomes a crucial component of improving health and ultimately extending a person's lifespan.

There are different strategies that you can use, and we focused on one particularly popular option in this book – intermittent fasting. In particular, we looked at how you can use the 16:8 intermittent fasting technique to help you shed excess body fat, while also building lean muscle mass and improving your overall body composition.

In addition to telling you how you can use the 16:8 intermittent fasting technique for weight loss, I also shared some highly effective and delicious meal options that you can use to ensure you can lose weight successfully while following this particular method of intermittent fasting.

From here, you can start to experiment with the meals that you include in your daily diet. There is no one-size-fits-all option when it comes to including a specific meal plan in your intermittent fasting plan. The guidance I provided you with here will help you better realize how you should get started.

Once you implement the meal plan that I discussed with you here, you should already be able to start experiencing the benefits that are associated with intermittent fasting. After a week or two, you'll be able to see if the diet helps you lose weight and make appropriate adjustments to the meal plan that you are following to better suit your needs, as well as the specific goals that you have in mind.

Decide if it is right for you. Even though there are some good benefits, remember IF is not for everyone. Your nutritional understanding and lifestyle exercise should determine if you are attempting IF. I strongly recommend that you first understand the essentials if you are new to exercise and nutrition. Begin with slowly, simply, and gradually. There is no rush if you decide you would like to try IF. Choose one little thing to try, even if it is just a one-hour regular meal adjustment. Try this and see how it is working for you. Concentrate on what IF approaches have in common, rather than getting too into detail. Sometimes you eat and sometimes you do not do it, that almost summarizes it.

Consider what is going on in your lives. Think about how much training you are doing and how intensively you are doing, how well you are resting and recovering, how well IF fits into your daily practice and ordinary personal operations, and what other pressure needs and life provide. Remember IF one of the many types of diet is that function. But it "works" only when it is constant, flexible, and parts of your normal practice, not a duty, and not a permanent trigger of physical and psychological stress.

Know yourself and observe your experiences carefully. Be an academic and start gathering data, gaining knowledge, and drawing conclusions that you use to guide future action. Do the right thing for you. You should also give yourself time. Especially since it usually takes a few weeks to adapt to your new program. Difficulties are expected; it is part of how life goes. It is life's element; they happen.

You need to be keenly conscious of how your body is responding to an ongoing program of fasting. Your body system will determine what you consume, how much time you consume, how much time you practice, how much calories you consume, etc. Considering all these variables will guarantee that you are in command of the program of fasting and, eventually, your weight.